AF412712

Tooth Movement

Frontiers of Oral Biology

Vol. 18

Series Editor

Paul T. Sharpe London

Tooth Movement

Volume Editors

Alpdogan Kantarci Cambridge, Mass.
Leslie Will Boston, Mass.
Stephen Yen Los Angeles, Calif.

57 figures, 16 in color, 2016

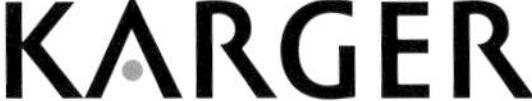

Basel · Freiburg · Paris · London · New York · Chennai · New Delhi · Bangkok · Beijing · Shanghai · Tokyo · Kuala Lumpur · Singapore · Sydney

Dr. Alpdogan Kantarci
The Forsyth Institute
Department of Applied Oral Sciences
245 First Street, #6103
Cambridge, MA 02142 (USA)

Dr. Stephen Yen
University of Southern California
Herman Ostrow School of Dentistry
Department of Orthodontics, Oral Surgery and
Basic Sciences
Los Angeles, CA (USA)

Dr. Leslie Will
Boston University
Henry M. Goldman School of Dental Medicine
Department of Orthodontics & Dentofacial Orthopedics
100 East Newton Street
Boston, MA 02118 (USA)

Library of Congress Cataloging-in-Publication Data

Tooth movement / volume editors, Alpdogan Kantarci, Leslie Will, Stephen Yen.
    p. ; cm. -- (Frontiers of oral biology, ISSN 1420-2433 ; vol. 18)
  Includes bibliographical references and indexes.
  ISBN 978-3-318-05479-8 (hard cover : alk. paper) -- ISBN 978-3-318-05480-4
(e-ISBN)
  I. Kantarci, Alpdogan, editor. II. Will, Leslie, editor. III. Yen, Stephen, editor. IV. Series: Frontiers of
oral biology ; v. 18. 1420-2433
  [DNLM: 1. Tooth Movement. W1 FR946GP v.18 2016 / WU 400]
  RK52
  362.1976--dc23

                                                    2015034833

Bibliographic Indices. This publication is listed in bibliographic services, including Current Contents® and Index Medicus.

© Copyright 2016 by S. Karger AG, P.O. Box, CH–4009 Basel (Switzerland)
www.karger.com
Printed in Germany on acid-free and non-aging paper (ISO 97069) by Kraft Druck GmbH, Ettlingen
ISSN 1420–2433
e-ISSN 1662–3770
ISBN 978–3–318–05479–8
e-ISBN 978–3–318–05480–4

Contents

Preface

We are privileged to have this opportunity to present this volume on the 'biology of tooth movement'. As the editors of this book, we aimed to cover various aspects of the biological basis and mechanisms of orthodontic tooth movement and the growing field of accelerated orthodontics. Enhancement of the rate, quality and stability of the orthodontic tooth movement has always been the goal of the practice. Many methods have been tried over the course of the last few decades with some of these techniques resulting in success. These approaches ranged from biologicals to mechanical stimulation and to surgical approaches with different invasiveness. The field is now moving towards accomplishing the 'acceleration' with less invasive or noninvasive methods. While the interest grows both at the clinical level and by the industry, the understanding of the biology is limited.

Valuable information has been gathered by the attempts over the past decades where we realized that a simple increase in force will result in tooth morbidity and the arrest of tooth migration. Another finding was that a multidisciplinary approach and teamwork were critical for success. New methods have been introduced and widely tested in humans, in animal models and in vitro; we have also recognized the importance of the translation of biological concepts into the clinical practice.

The twenty-first century is the era of 'omics'. Biology and complex interactions between systems are not anymore limited to single-molecule testing only and associations with a physiological process. Diseases and functions are related and present a complex network of events, which include genomics, proteomics, lipidomics and transcriptomics. In the oral cavity, these events take place in an environment heavily colonized by the largest body of bacterial species in humans introducing the microbiome. Meanwhile, no other part of the mammalian system has been exposed to the complex biomechanical forces regulated by hormones and neurons as in the oral cavity and in the periodontal ligament. This challenging but exciting era introduces novel ideas and requires an integration of science and clinical applications. Orthodontics is certainly not exempt from these innovations; dentoalveolar structures are bathed in microbes, biomechanics impact almost every cell type and process, and the clinical outcomes are determined by the biological variations.

This volume presents a multidisciplinary expertise on a wide variety of processes related to and involved in orthodontic tooth movement. The premise was that by a better understanding of the biological structures and the mechanism through which they respond to biomechanical forces, one can get a better perspective on the 'acceleration'. Recent data demonstrate that different pathways of activation may be involved in accelerated orthodontic tooth movement compared to the conventional approaches. It is critical to understand which mechanisms are being involved related to the biology and metabolism of alveolar bone. The first section in the book focuses on the periodontal ligament as well as cellular and molecular aspects of bone remodeling under physiological and pathological conditions. The second section presents the mechanical properties of dentoalveolar structures as the two major concepts of regional acceleratory phenomenon and biomechanics. Third, orthodontic tooth movement is discussed from a historical perspective and as the basis for stability and relapse while emerging concepts of neurological regulation and coupling between osteoclasts and osteoblasts are presented. The last section is devoted to the various approaches for accelerating the orthodontic tooth movement. Each section has been authored by experts in this exciting field of great interest for both the academician and the clinician.

The strength of the volume is the body of internationally recognized expert contributors and their outstanding work. As editors, we highly appreciate those who made this book possible. The concept of this text was conceived based on the notion that there is a need for a nontextbook compilation of research in accelerated orthodontics. This field is developing fast, and we are fully aware that new research will change many paradigms. The goal of this book is to present the recent advances with the hope that future research will take full advantage of the changes in clinical practice based on the biological bases.

Alpdogan Kantarci, Cambridge, Mass.
Stephen Yen, Los Angeles, Calif.
Leslie A. Will, Boston, Mass.

Kantarci A, Will L, Yen S (eds): Tooth Movement. Front Oral Biol. Basel, Karger, 2016, vol 18, pp 1–8
DOI: 10.1159/000351894

Periodontal Ligament and Alveolar Bone in Health and Adaptation: Tooth Movement

Nan Jiang · Weihua Guo · Mo Chen · Ying Zheng · Jian Zhou ·
Sahng Gyoon Kim · Mildred C. Embree · Karen Songhee Song ·
Heloisa F. Marao · Jeremy J. Mao

Center for Craniofacial Regeneration, Columbia University Medical Center, New York, N.Y., USA

Abstract

The periodontal ligament (PDL) and alveolar bone are two critical tissues for understanding orthodontic tooth movement. The current literature is replete with descriptive studies of multiple cell types and their matrices in the PDL and alveolar bone, but is deficient with how stem/progenitor cells differentiate into PDL and alveolar bone cells. Can one type of orthodontic force with a specific magnitude and frequency activate osteoblasts, whereas another force type activates osteoclasts? This chapter will discuss the biology of not only mature cells and their matrices in the periodontal ligament and alveolar bone, but also stem/progenitor cells that differentiate into fibroblasts, osteoblasts and osteoclasts. Key advances in tooth movement rely on further understanding of osteoblast and fibroblast differentiation from mesenchymal stem/progenitor cells, and osteoclastogenesis from the hematopoietic/monocyte lineage.   © 2016 S. Karger AG, Basel

The alveolar bone, periodontal ligament (PDL) and cementum are intimately related structures in development and functions. Collectively, they form the periodontium that is of critical relevance not only to orthodontic tooth movement, but also

periodontal disease. There are myriads of descriptive studies of multiple cell types and their gene expression profiles of the PDL and alveolar bone, often separately in orthodontics and periodontal research literatures. Matrix synthesis is another area of focus of numerous investigations of the PDL and alveolar bone. Far deficient is our understanding of how stem/progenitor cells differentiate into mature cells in the PDL and alveolar bone, including fibroblasts, osteoblasts and osteoclasts [1]. This deficiency applies to not only our understanding in homeostasis, but also as adaptive responses during tooth movement and periodontal disease.

This chapter focuses on three related topics: (1) fundamental cell and matrix structures of the PDL and alveolar bone, (2) PDL and alveolar bone remodeling during orthodontics tooth movement, and (3) how our understanding of PDL and alveolar bone stem/progenitor cells may help advance orthodontics. Orthodontic tooth movement is typically divided into three phases by clinical observation: the initial phase, the lag phase, and the postlag phase [2]. The initial phase occurs 24–48 h after force application. The lag phase lasts multiple days with little tooth movement. The post-lag phase is when clinically noticeable tooth movement is observed. To date, our understanding of how stem/progenitor cells are involved in orthodontic tooth movement remains at an infancy stage.

Periodontal Ligament

The PDL connects the cementum to the alveolar bone by bundles of type I collagen named Sharpey's fibers. The width of a periodontal ligament in homeostasis is approximately 0.15–0.38 mm, depending on the tooth type. The PDL has two primary functions: (1) to transmit and absorb mechanical stress and (2) to provide vascular supply and nutrients to the cementum, alveolar bone and the PDL itself [3]. The PDL is a connective tissue and shares certain similarities with tendons and other ligaments in the appendicular skeleton [4].

Cells
Fibroblasts constitute about 50–60% of the total PDL cellularity [5]. PDL fibroblasts consist of multiple subpopulations and thus are heterogeneous. PDL cells experience and respond to mechanical stresses [6], such as those in orthodontic tooth movement. Other PDL cells include macrophages, lymphocytes and endothelial cells that form the lining of blood vessels [7]. When forces are applied to the tooth, PDL fibroblasts react by activating stretch-sensitive Ca^{2+}-permeable channels and increase actin polymerization and yield a rapid and transient increase in c-fos expression that in turn stimulates their proliferation and differentiation [8]. Activated fibroblasts secrete plasminogen activator as well as its inhibitor, matrix metalloproteases and their inhibitors, cytokines (PGE-2) and interleukin-6 [9].

The PDL further consists of defense cells such as macrophages and mast cells. Epithelial remnants of Malassez are descents of dental epithelium cells in the PDL, following amelogenesis. In addition, osteoblasts, osteoclasts and cementoblasts are present in the PDL and participate in the homeostasis of the periodontium. The osteoblasts and osteoclasts reside in the PDL on the surface of lamina dura and in endosteal surfaces of the alveolar bone, and are also responsive to mechanical stresses.

PDL and alveolar bone readily remodel in homeostasis and orthodontic tooth movement. Osteoblasts in the PDL and alveolar bone are replaced every few months [10]. Most biological tissues adapt and self-renew, serving as an indication that there must be stem cells, which replenish and replace terminally differentiated cells that periodically undergo apoptosis. Stem cells are immature and unspecialized cells that can (1) self-renew and (2) undergo asymmetrical differentiation: producing precise copies of stem cells and at the same time differentiate into specialized cell types such as fibroblasts and osteoblasts. In a developing embryo, embryonic stem cells can differentiate into every single 200 types of specialized cells in the body, and therefore, are called pluripotent stem cells [11]. In the adult, stem cells are likely more restricted and can differentiate into a limited number of cell types, but nonetheless, can replenish mature cells that are lost to apoptosis [12]. Postnatal stem/progenitor cells are more restricted in the number of lineages that they can differentiate into. Typically, progenitor cells differentiate into only one type of mature cells during homeostasis.

There are two types of dental stem cells: epithelial stem cells and mesenchymal stem cells [13, 14]. Epithelial and mesenchymal stem cells intimately interact during tooth development: epithelial stem cells giving rise to ameloblasts, whereas mesenchymal stem cells differentiating into fibroblasts, odontoblasts, cementoblasts, osteoblasts, and perhaps other cells in the periodontal ligament [15].

Periodontal ligament cells have been studied for decades, due to their significance in periodontal disease and also orthodontic tooth movement. Dental follicle cells, which originate from neural crest derived mesenchyme, differentiate into cells that form the periodontium and are present in the developing tooth germ prior to root formation [16]. Among fibroblast-like cells in the periodontal ligament, stem/progenitor cells have been identified [17]. Typically, soft tissue is scraped from the root of an extracted tooth and enzyme-digested to release a small number of cells. Morphologically, it is impossible to separate PDL fibroblasts from PDL stem/progenitor cells. Nonetheless, certain PDL cells yield progenies upon single cell colony assay and can differentiate into multiple cell lineages in vitro. In chemically defined culture conditions, specific PDL cells differentiate into cementoblast-like cells, adipocytes, and collagen-forming cells. When transplanted into immune-compromised rodents, PDL fibroblast-like cells generated a cementum/PDL-like structure [17]. To date, little is known how PDL stem/progenitor cells respond to mechanical forces such as those in orthodontic tooth movement.

Fibrous Matrix
Collagen fibers, reticulin fibers and oxytalan fibers form the PDL fibrous matrix. Collagen accounts for over 90% PDL fibers. Type I collagen fibers in the PDL are 45–55 nm in diameter and have somewhat uniform morphology [18]. PDL fiber bundles are arranged in directions that reflect their functional properties. PDL collagen fibers grow separately from bone and cementum surfaces, and gradually elongate and approximate each other [19].

Upon application of orthodontic forces, PDL nerve fibers release calcitonin gene-related peptide (CGRP) and substance P [20]. CGRP and substance P serve as vasodilators and stimulate plasma extravasation and leukocyte migration. CGRP has been shown to induce bone formation through stimulation of osteoblasts and inhibition of osteoclast activity [21].

Alveolar Bone

A better name for the alveolar bone is dental bone or tooth bone, for tooth loss leads to disappearance of the alveolar bone. Although the bulk of the alveolar bone is trabecular bone, it does contain a plate of compact bone adjacent to the periodontal ligament called the lamina dura. The PDL pierces through the lamina dura and anchors to the alveolar bone, with the other end connected to the cementum [22]. The inner (lingual) and outer (labial) cortical plates are also composed of compact bone.

Alveolar bone is a mineralized connective tissue and consists of mineral tissue, organic matrix and water. In the alveolar bone, 23% is mineralized tissue; 37% is the organic matrix which mostly is collagen, and the other 40% is water [23].

Cells
Multiple cell types are responsible for the homeostasis and functions of the alveolar bone. The most obvious cell types are osteoblasts, osteocytes and osteoclasts. However, other cell types are also important, including adipocytes, endothelial cells that form the lining of blood vessels and immune competent cells such as macrophages.

Osteoblasts are mononucleated and specialized cells that are responsible for bone apposition. Osteoblasts and fibroblasts share a key functional similarity in that they both synthesize type I collagen matrix. Osteoblasts, however, distinguish from fibroblasts by expressing Cbfa1 or Runx2 that is a master switch for the differentiation of stem/progenitor cells into osteoblasts [24]. Although myriad genes control the complex process of osteogenesis, Cbfa1 or Runx2 is the earliest transcriptional factor and signals the initiation of bone formation [25]. Other osteogenesis genes include bone morphogenetic proteins, transforming growth factor-β, Indian hedgehog and ostrix [26–29]. Bone is a dynamic tissue and constantly remodels by osteoblasts and osteoclasts, the two of which function by cross talk and signaling [25]. The number of osteoblasts decreases with age, affecting the balance of bone deposition and resorption and potentially leading to osteoporosis [30].

Mesenchymal stem/progenitor cells have been isolated from jaw bones of both humans and rodents [31–33]. Stem/progenitor cells from the jaw bone were clonogenic and had potent osteogenic potential in vitro and in vivo [33]. Compared with iliac crest cells, mandibular mesenchymal stem/progenitor cells appear to proliferate rapidly with delayed senescence, express robust alkaline phosphatase and accumulate more calcium in vitro [31]. Specifically, mesenchymal stem/progenitor cells from long bones yield greater bone marrow area than mandibular mesenchymal stem/progenitor cells when transplanted heterotopically in vivo [32].

Osteocytes are the most numerous cells in mature bone, and can live as long as the organism itself [34]. Osteocytes are derived from functional osteoblasts that are embedded in mineralized bone in the process of bone apposition. The space that an osteocyte occupies is called a lacuna. Hydroxyapatite, calcium carbonate and calcium phosphate is deposited around osteocytes [35, 36].

Whereas osteoblasts (and osteocytes) derive from the mesenchymal/mesodermal lineage, osteoclasts originate from an entirely different source: the hematopoietic/monocyte lineage [37, 38]. Osteoclasts are formed by the fusion of multiple monocytes, and, therefore, multinucleated [39, 40]. Their unique properties include adherence to endosteal bone surfaces, and secret acid and lytic enzymes that destroy mineral and protein structures. An array of transcription factors controls osteoclast differentiation [40]. Osteoclasts are characterized by robust expression of tartrate resistant acid phosphatase, specified osteoprotegerin, cathepsin K, and chloride channel 7 (ClCN7) [41]. Osteoprotegerin blocks nuclear factor-kappa B (RANK) and RANK ligand (RANKL) docking; cathepsin K destroys bone matrix proteins, whereas chloride channel 7 maintains osteoclast neutrality by shuffling chloride ions through the cell membrane. RANKL, a key regulator of osteoclast function [39, 40], is synthesized by osteoblasts and promotes osteoclast differentiation, suggesting that osteoblasts control osteoclast differentiation, but not function [42].

Matrix Proteins

In the alveolar bone, the most abundant extracellular matrix component is collagen type I [43]. In addition, alveolar bone contains noncollagenous proteins such as osteocalcin, osteopontin, osteonectin, bone sialoprotein and fibronectin as well as proteoglycans including lumican, fibromodulin, decorin, biglycan and versican. Osteocalcin acts as a hormone and causes pancreatic beta cells to release more insulin, and at the same time directs adipocytes to release adiponectin, which increases sensitivity to insulin [44]. Osteopontin is a phosphorylated, sialic acid containing glycoprotein that can be extracted from the mineralized bone matrix. Matrix metalloproteinase-1, metalloproteinase-2 [43, 45] and cathepsin [46, 47] are considered to be particularly important in bone resorption. They cleave type I collagen most efficiently within the triple-helical body of the native conformation and is active at neutral pH, whereas cathepsin K degrades type I collagen in a similar manner but is active at low pH in the acidic microenvironment beneath the ruffled border of osteoclasts [48].

Periodontal Ligament and Alveolar Bone Resorption and Remodeling

Can one type of force with a specific magnitude and frequency preferably activate osteoblasts, whereas another force type preferably activates osteoclasts [49]. One can only begin to address a question such as this by understanding how stem/progenitor cells in the PDL and alveolar differentiate into mature cells, including fibroblasts, osteoblasts, osteoclasts and endothelial cells. Two interrelated processes in orthodontic tooth movement are deflection (bending) of the alveolar bone and remodeling of the periodontium: the periodontal ligament, alveolar bone and cementum [50]. In the 'pressure-tension theory', the PDL senses a change in mechanical forces or stresses. The theory proposes that PDL progenitor cells differentiate into compression-associated osteoclasts and tension-associated osteoblasts, causing bone resorption and apposition, respectively [51]. The following biological processes are proposed on the compression side: disturbance of blood flow in the compressed PDL, cell death in the compressed area of the PDL (hyalinization), resorption of the hyalinized tissue by macrophages, and undermining bone resorption by osteoclasts beside the hyalinized tissue. It is proposed that tooth movement follows the completion of these processes on the compression side, but not before.

On the tension side, it is proposed that the periodontium, including the PDL, alveolar bone and cementum remodels and undergoes bone apposition. Osteoblasts differentiate from mesenchymal stem/progenitor cells. Mature osteoblasts form the osteoid or type I collagen matrix, which is followed by mineralization [52]. Endothelial nitric oxide synthase mediates bone formation on the tension side of orthodontic forces [53].

Force magnitude has been associated with biological events, although most of these associations are conjectures. 'Direct resorption' is associated with light force application, tissue and cell preservation, and vascular potency. 'Indirect resorption' and hyalinization are associated with heavy forces that cause crushing injury to PDL tissues, cell death, hemostasis, and cell-free PDL and adjacent alveolar bone zones [54]. Mechanical forces often cause hyalinization leading to necrosis in the PDL and lead to delayed bone resorption. Hyalinization occurs in the PDL and is proposed to indicate hyaline-like tissue forma-

tion that no longer has normal tissue architecture. Macrophages are responsible for removing the hyalinized tissues prior to which little tooth movement occurs [55]. Extracellular matrix and cell distortion causes structural and functional changes in cell membrane, and cytoskeletal proteins. At the same time, numerous submembrane proteins associate in cellular focal adhesions. These complex structural or functional adaptations will transmit signals to the cytoplasm and mediate cell adhesion by integrin activation [56].

Alveolar bone resorption occurs on the compression side during tooth movement. Bone resorption occurs through osteoclastic activity, thus creating irregular cavities in bone that later will be filled by newly formed bone owing to osteoblast activity. Two processes involved in bone resorption are the dissolution of minerals and the degradation of the organ matrix, which consists of type I collagen. These processes are driven by enzymes, including matrix metalloproteinase and lysosome cysteine proteinases [48]. Orthodontic forces result in the deformation of blood vessels and disarrangement of surrounding tissues. Subsequently, blood flow and periodontal tissue adapt to the compression force, or when they fail, are responsible for cell death and tissue necrosis [57].

The rate of orthodontic tooth movement is affected by multiple factors such as the magnitude, frequency, and duration of mechanical forces that are applied to the teeth or bone. Mechanical forces change vascularity and blood flow, resulting in the synthesis and release of molecules such as neurotransmitters, cytokines, growth factors, colony-stimulating factors that regulate leucocyte, macrophage, and monocyte lines [58, 59].

Protein phosphorylation mediated by protein kinase enzymes is critical to the understanding of orthodontic tooth movement [56, 60, 61]. Cytoplasmic signaling proteins Hh, sonic hedge-hog, the transforming growth factor-β superfamily, and many transcription factors and ions

(Ca^{2+}, PO^{3-}) enhance or suppress gene expression. Matrix metalloproteinases (MMP) is an indispensable enzyme in bone remodeling. MMP-2 protein is induced by compression and increases significantly in a time-dependent fashion, reaching a peak after 8 h of force application. On the tension side, MMP-2 significantly increases after one hour of force application but gradually returns to baseline within eight hours [62]. The cleavages of procollagen yields procollagen type I C-terminal propeptide and procollagen type I N-terminal propeptide that may serve as bone formation markers [63]. Normal chloride channels play a key role in osteoclastic alveolar bone resorption in orthodontic tooth movement [40]. Cystic fibrosis, a pathological bone condition is characterized by mutated cellular chloride channels encoded by polymorphic nucleotide sequences in the ClCN7 gene [50].

ing mechanical stresses to biochemical events with a net result of bone apposition and/or bone resorption. Despite our improved understanding of mechanical and biochemical signaling mechanisms, how mechanical stresses regulate the differentiation of stem/progenitor cells into osteoblast lineage and osteoclast lineage is largely unknown. An improved understanding of osteoblast differentiation from mesenchymal stem/progenitor cells and osteoclastogenesis from the hematopoietic/monocyte lineage is essential to advance orthodontics. Design of orthodontic force systems has been largely empirical since the Angle era. The orthodontics community is now equipped with tools to begin advancing the understanding of orthodontic tooth movement via cellular and molecular events, including how stem cells differentiate into osteoblasts and osteoclasts.

Conclusion

The periodontal ligament and alveolar bone make up a functional unit and undergo robust remodeling in orthodontic tooth movement. Complex molecular signaling is responsible for transduc-

Acknowledgements

The authors wish to thank F. Guo, H. Keyes and J. Melendez for technical and administrative assistance. The effort for composition of this article is supported by NIH grants R01DE018248, R01EB009663, and RC2DE020767 to J.J. Mao.

References

1 Mao JJ, Robey PG, Prockop DJ: Stem cells in the face: tooth regeneration and beyond. Cell Stem Cell 2012;11:291–301.

2 Krishnan V, Davidovitch Z: Cellular, molecular, and tissue-level reactions to orthodontic force. Am J Orthod Dentofacial Orthop 2006;129:469.e461–e432.

3 Storey E: The nature of tooth movement. Am J Orthod 1973;63:292–314.

4 Nanci A, Bosshardt DD: Structure of periodontal tissues in health and disease. Periodontol 2000 2006;40:11–28.

5 McCulloch CA, Bordin S: Role of fibroblast subpopulations in periodontal physiology and pathology. J Periodontal Res 1991;26:144–154.

6 Phipps RP, Borrello MA, Blieden TM: Fibroblast heterogeneity in the periodontium and other tissues. J Periodontal Res 1997;32:159–165.

7 Naveh GR, Lev-Tov Chattah N, Zaslansky P, Shahar R, Weiner S: Tooth-PDL-bone complex: Response to compressive loads encountered during mastication. A review. Arch Oral Biol 2012;57:1575–1584.

8 Yamaguchi N, Chiba M, Mitani H: The induction of c-fos mRNA expression by mechanical stress in human periodontal ligament cells. Arch Oral Biol 2002;47:465–471.

9 Lekic PC, Rajshankar D, Chen H, Tenenbaum H, McCulloch CA: Transplantation of labeled periodontal ligament cells promotes regeneration of alveolar bone. Anat Rec 2001;262:193–202.

10 Davidovitch Z: Tooth movement. Crit Rev Oral Biol Med 1991;2:411–450.

11 Boyer LA, Lee TI, Cole MF, Johnstone SE, Levine SS, Zucker JP, Guenther MG, Kumar RM, Murray HL, Jenner RG, et al: Core transcriptional regulatory circuitry in human embryonic stem cells. Cell 2005;122:947–956.

12 Scholer HR: The potential of stem cells. A status update. Bundesgesundheitsblatt Gesundheitsforsch Gesundheitsschutz 2004;47:565–577.

13   Harada H, Kettunen P, Jung HS, Mustonen T, Wang YA, Thesleff I: Localization of putative stem cells in dental epithelium and their association with Notch and FGF signaling. J Cell Biol 1999;147:105–120.

14   Sonoyama W, Liu Y, Fang DAJ, Yamaza T, Seo BM, Zhang CM, Liu H, Gronthos S, Wang CY, Shi ST, et al: Mesenchymal stem cell-mediated functional tooth regeneration in swine. Plos One 2006; 1:e79.

15   Bluteau G, Luder HU, De Bari C, Mitsiadis TA: Stem cells for tooth engineering. Eur Cells Mater 2008;16:1–9.

16   Yao S, Pan F, Prpic V, Wise GE: Differentiation of stem cells in the dental follicle. J Dent Res 2008;87:767–771.

17   Seo BM, Miura M, Gronthos S, Bartold PM, Batouli S, Brahim J, Young M, Robey PG, Wang CY, Shi S: Investigation of multipotent postnatal stem cells from human periodontal ligament. Lancet 2004;364:149–155.

18   MacNeill S, Walters DM, Dey A, Glaros AG, Cobb CM: Sonic and mechanical toothbrushes. An in vitro study showing altered microbial surface structures but lack of effect on viability. J Clin Periodontol 1998;25:988–993.

19   Sawhney RK, Howard J: Molecular dissection of the fibroblast-traction machinery. Cell Motil Cytoskel 2004;58: 175–185.

20   Hall M, Masella R, Meister M: PDL neuron-associated neurotransmitters in orthodontic tooth movement: identification and proposed mechanism of action. Today's FDA 2001;13:24–25.

21   Anderson LE, Seybold VS: Calcitonin gene-related peptide regulates gene transcription in primary afferent neurons. J Neurochem 2004;91:1417–1429.

22   Blum IR: Contemporary views on dry socket (alveolar osteitis): a clinical appraisal of standardization, aetiopathogenesis and management: a critical review. Int J Oral Maxillofac Surg 2002;31: 309–317.

23   Moss-Salentijn L: Melvin L: Moss and the functional matrix. J Dent Res 1997; 76:1814–1817.

24   Ehrlich PJ, Lanyon LE: Mechanical strain and bone cell function: a review. Osteoporos Int 2002;13:688–700.

25   Ducy P, Schinke T, Karsenty G: The osteoblast: a sophisticated fibroblast under central surveillance. Science 2000;289: 1501–1504.

26   Winkler DG, Sutherland MK, Geoghegan JC, Yu CP, Hayes T, Skonier JE, Shpektor D, Jonas M, Kovacevich BR, Staehling-Hampton K, et al: Osteocyte control of bone formation via sclerostin, a novel BMP antagonist. Embo J 2003; 22:6267–6276.

27   Mackie EJ: Osteoblasts: novel roles in orchestration of skeletal architecture. Int J Biochem Cell B 2003;35:1301–1305.

28   Bu RF, Borysenko CW, Li YN, Cao LH, Sabokbar A, Blair HC: Expression and function of TNF-family proteins and receptors in human osteoblasts. Bone 2003;33:760–770.

29   Ducy P, Schinke T, Karsenty G: The osteoblast: a sophisticated fibroblast under central surveillance. Science 2000;289: 1501–1504.

30   D'Ippolito G, Schiller PC, Ricordi C, Roos BA, Howard GA: Age-related osteogenic potential of mesenchymal stromal stem cells from human vertebral bone marrow. J Bone Miner Res 1999; 14:1115–1122.

31   Akintoye SO, Lam T, Shi S, Brahim J, Collins MT, Robey PG: Skeletal site-specific characterization of orofacial and iliac crest human bone marrow stromal cells in same individuals. Bone 2006;38: 758–768.

32   Yamaza T, Ren G, Akiyama K, Chen C, Shi Y, Shi S: Mouse mandible contains distinctive mesenchymal stem cells. J Dent Res 2011;90:317–324.

33   Matsubara T, Suardita K, Ishii M, Sugiyama M, Igarashi A, Oda R, Nishimura M, Saito M, Nakagawa K, Yamanaka K, et al: Alveolar bone marrow as a cell source for regenerative medicine: differences between alveolar and iliac bone marrow stromal cells. J Bone Miner Res 2005;20:399–409.

34   Mullender MG, van der Meer DD, Huiskes R, Lips P: Osteocyte density changes in aging and osteoporosis. Bone 1996; 18:109–113.

35   Noble BS: The osteocyte lineage. Arch Biochem Biophys 2008;473:106–111.

36   Marotti G, Ferretti M, Muglia MA, Palumbo C, Palazzini S: A quantitative-evaluation of osteoblast-osteocyte relationships on growing endosteal surface of rabbit tibiae. Bone 1992;13:363–368.

37   Nijweide PJ, Burger EH, Feyen JH: Cells of bone: proliferation, differentiation, and hormonal regulation. Physiol Rev 1986;66:855–886.

38   Holtrop ME, King GJ: The ultrastructure of the osteoclast and its functional implications. Clin Orthop Relat Res 1977; 123:177–196.

39   Boyle WJ, Simonet WS, Lacey DL: Osteoclast differentiation and activation. Nature 2003;423:337–342.

40   Teitelbaum SL: Bone resorption by osteoclasts. Science 2000;289:1504–1508.

41   Harada S, Rodan GA: Control of osteoblast function and regulation of bone mass. Nature 2003;423:349–355.

42   Karsenty G: The complexities of skeletal biology. Nature 2003;423:316–318.

43   Delaisse JM, Eeckhout Y, Neff L, Francois-Gillet C, Henriet P, Su Y, Vaes G, Baron R: (Pro)collagenase (matrix metalloproteinase-1) is present in rodent osteoclasts and in the underlying bone-resorbing compartment. J Cell Sci 1993; 106:1071–1082.

44   Lee NK, Sowa H, Hinoi E, Ferron M, Ahn JD, Confavreux C, Dacquin R, Mee PJ, McKee MD, Jung DY, et al: Endocrine regulation of energy metabolism by the skeleton. Cell 2007;130: 456–469.

45   Chambers TJ, Revell PA, Fuller K, Athanasou NA: Resorption of bone by isolated rabbit osteoclasts. J Cell Sci 1984; 66:383–399.

46   Drake FH, Dodds RA, James IE, Connor JR, Debouck C, Richardson S, Lee-Rykaczewski E, Coleman L, Rieman D, Barthlow R, et al: Cathepsin K, but not cathepsins B, L, or S, is abundantly expressed in human osteoclasts. J Biol Chem 1996;271:12511–12516.

47   Bossard MJ, Tomaszek TA, Thompson SK, Amegadzie BY, Hanning CR, Jones C, Kurdyla JT, McNulty DE, Drake FH, Gowen M, et al: Proteolytic activity of human osteoclast cathepsin K. Expression, purification, activation, and substrate identification. J Biol Chem 1996; 271:12517–12524.

48   Domon S, Shimokawa H, Matsumoto Y, Yamaguchi S, Soma K: In situ hybridization for matrix metalloproteinase-1 and cathepsin K in rat root-resorbing tissue induced by tooth movement. Arch Oral Biol 1999;44:907–915.

49   Mao JJ: Orthodontics at a pivotal point of transformation. Semin Orthodont 2010;16:143–146.

50   Masella RS, Meister M: Current concepts in the biology of orthodontic tooth movement. Am J Orthod Dentofacial Orthop 2006;129:458–468.

51 Henneman S, Von den Hoff JW, Maltha JC: Mechanobiology of tooth movement. Eur J Orthod 2008;30:299–306.

52 Sprogar S, Vaupotic T, Cor A, Drevensek M, Drevensek G: The endothelin system mediates bone modeling in the late stage of orthodontic tooth movement in rats. Bone 2008;43:740–747.

53 Tan SD, Xie R, Klein-Nulend J, van Rheden RE, Bronckers AL, Kuijpers-Jagtman AM, Von den Hoff JW, Maltha JC: Orthodontic force stimulates eNOS and iNOS in rat osteocytes. J Dent Res 2009;88:255–260.

54 Brudvik P, Rygh P: The repair of orthodontic root resorption: an ultrastructural study. Eur J Orthod 1995;17:189–198.

55 von Bohl M, Maltha JC, Von Den Hoff JW, Kuijpers-Jagtman AM: Focal hyalinization during experimental tooth movement in beagle dogs. Am J Orthod Dentofacial Orthop 2004;125:615–623.

56 McLean GW, Komiyama NH, Serrels B, Asano H, Reynolds L, Conti F, Hodivala-Dilke K, Metzger D, Chambon P, Grant SG, et al: Specific deletion of focal adhesion kinase suppresses tumor formation and blocks malignant progression. Genes Dev 2004;18:2998–3003.

57 Kitase Y, Yokozeki M, Fujihara S, Izawa T, Kuroda S, Tanimoto K, Moriyama K, Tanaka E: Analysis of gene expression profiles in human periodontal ligament cells under hypoxia: the protective effect of CC chemokine ligand 2 to oxygen shortage. Arch Oral Biol 2009;54:618–624.

58 Zainal Ariffin SH, Yamamoto Z, Zainol Abidin IZ, Megat Abdul Wahab R, Zainal Ariffin Z: Cellular and molecular changes in orthodontic tooth movement. Sci World J 2011;11:1788–1803.

59 Bartzela T, Turp JC, Motschall E, Maltha JC: Medication effects on the rate of orthodontic tooth movement: a systematic literature review. Am J Orthod Dentofacial Orthop 2009;135:16–26.

60 York JD, Hunter T: Signal transduction. Unexpected mediators of protein phosphorylation. Science 2004;306:2053–2055.

61 Bettencourt-Dias M, Giet R, Sinka R, Mazumdar A, Lock WG, Balloux F, Zafiropoulos PJ, Yamaguchi S, Winter S, Carthew RW, et al: Genome-wide survey of protein kinases required for cell cycle progression. Nature 2004;432:980–987.

62 Cantarella G, Cantarella R, Caltabiano M, Risuglia N, Bernardini R, Leonardi R: Levels of matrix metalloproteinases 1 and 2 in human gingival crevicular fluid during initial tooth movement. Am J Orthod Dentofacial Orthop 2006;130:568.e511–e566.

63 Hannon RA, Eastell R: Bone markers and current laboratory assays. Cancer Treat Rev 2006;32(suppl 1):7–14.

Jeremy J. Mao, DDS, PhD
Center for Craniofacial Regeneration, Columbia University Medical Center
630 W. 168 St. – PH7E – CDM
New York, NY 10032 (USA)
E-Mail jmao@columbia.edu

Jiang · Guo · Chen · Zheng · Zhou · Kim · Embree · Songhee Song · Marao · Mao

Kantarci A, Will L, Yen S (eds): Tooth Movement. Front Oral Biol. Basel, Karger, 2016, vol 18, pp 9–16
DOI: 10.1159/000351895

Cellular and Molecular Aspects of Bone Remodeling

Wenmei Xiao[a, d] · Yu Wang[c, d] · Sandra Pacios[d, e] · Shuai Li[b, d] · Dana T. Graves[d]

Departments of [a]Periodontology and [b]Implantology, School and Hospital of Stomatology, Peking University, Beijing, and [c]Department of Dental Implantology, School and Hospital of Stomatology, Jilin University, Jilin, China; [d]Department of Periodontics, School of Dental Medicine, University of Pennsylvania, Philadelphia, Pa., USA; [e]Department of Periodontology, School of Dental Medicine, Universitat Internacional de 29 Catalunya, Sant Cugat del Vallès, Spain

Abstract

Bone remodeling is a highly coordinated process responsible for bone resorption and formation. It is initiated and modulated by a number of factors including inflammation, changes in hormonal levels and lack of mechanical stimulation. Bone remodeling involves the removal of mineralized bone by osteoclasts followed by the formation of bone matrix through osteoblasts that subsequently becomes mineralized. In addition to the traditional bone cells (osteoclasts, osteoblasts and osteocytes) that are necessary for bone remodeling, several immune cells such as polymorphonuclear neutrophils, B cells and T cells have also been implicated in bone remodelling. Through the receptor activator of nuclear factor-κB/receptor activator of the NF-κB ligand/osteoprotegerin system the process of bone resorption is initiated and subsequent formation is tightly coupled. Mediators such as prostaglandins, interleukins, chemokines, leukotrienes, growth factors, wnt signalling and bone morphogenetic proteins are involved in the regulation of bone remodeling. We discuss here cells and mediators involved in the cellular and molecular machanisms of bone resorption and bone formation.

© 2016 S. Karger AG, Basel

Cell Types Involved in Bone Remodeling

Bone remodeling is a lifelong process where old bone is removed (resorption) and new bone is created (formation) [1, 2]. This process is regulated by different cell types that form bone (osteoblasts), regulate bone homeostasis (osteocytes), resorb bone (osteoclasts) and affect bone resorption and formation (innate and adaptive immune cells). There are several pathologic processes that can affect bone remodeling whereby both bone resorption and formation are affected and have been demonstrated in post-menopausal osteoporosis, arthritis, periodontal disease and microgravity or disuse [2].

Osteoclasts are terminally differentiated myeloid cells that are uniquely adapted to remove mineralized bone matrix [1]. They are found in pits within the bone surface which are called resorption bays, also known as Howship's Lacunae. Osteoclasts resorb bone by producing acid that dissolves the mineral content and enzymes that remove the organic matrix. Mature osteoclasts anchor to the bone through RGD-binding sites to create a sealed microenvironment.

Osteoblasts are bone-forming cells that arise from osteoprogenitor cells. RUNX2 (runt-related transcription factor 2) and other transcription factors control the differentiation of osteoblasts [2–4]. During bone formation, a subpopulation of osteoblasts undergoes terminal differentiation and becomes engulfed by osteoid, at which time they are referred to as osteoid osteocytes. Osteocytes which reside in lacunae are the most numerous cell type found in mature bone and are long-lived. They have dendritic processes that interact with other osteocytes and bone-lining cells on the bone surface. Osteocytes respond to mechanical load. Under resting conditions osteocytes express sclerostin, which directly prevents Wnt signaling (described in more detail below). Sclerostin expression can be inhibited by parathyroid hormone signaling to remove this inhibitor of Wnt signaling and allow Wnt directed bone formation to occur. Under basal conditions, osteocytes secrete transforming growth factor β (TGF-β), which inhibits osteoclastogenesis. However, upon stimulation osteoblasts and osteocytes produce osteoclastogenic factors such as macrophage colony-stimulating factor-1 (CSF-1) and receptor activator of the NF-κB ligand (RANKL) to induce bone remodeling [1–4].

Innate immune cells (primarily polymorphonuclear neutrophils (PMNS), monocytes/macrophages and dendritic cells) and adaptive immune cells (primarily lymphocytes) modulate bone resorption particularly under inflammatory conditions. PMNs are granular leukocytes that predominate in the initial acute inflammatory response. Like other leukocytes, they are recruited from the peripheral vasculature by chemotactic factors, particularly chemokines. They express a number of inflammatory cytokines (e.g. IL-1β, TNF-α, IL-6) as well as membrane-bound RANKL [4]. Macrophages are produced from the differentiation of monocytes in tissue. Monocytes/macrophages can have an inflammatory or a pro-vascularization phenotype called M1 or M2. M1 macrophages produce cytokines such as IL-1β, TNF-α and RANKL, whereas M2 monocytes/macrophages produce anti-inflammatory mediators such as IL-10 and IL-4 [5]. Dendritic immune cells have their origin in bone marrow and are found in a number of different tissues. One of the first contacts between oral bacteria and the immune system occurs with Langerhans cells, a subset of dendritic cells found in mucosal surfaces and skin. They function in activating the immune response as antigen presenting cells and regulate homeostasis by modulating the response to oral bacteria and self-antigens. Once they detect antigen dendritic cells travel to lymph nodes and present antigen to activate lymphocytes.

The predominant cells of the adaptive immune response are B and T lymphocytes. Activated T and B cells can express RANKL and various other cytokines that typically promote osteoclastogenesis. B cells express TNF-α, IL-6, and RANKL to promote osteoclastogenesis. T cells can develop into T-helper cells, Th1, Th2 and Th17 that modulate bone resorption. Th1-type produce IL-1 and TNF-α that can promote bone resorption. Th17 cells have recently been identified as an effector T helper cell subset characterized by the production of proinflammatory cytokines. IL-1 and IL-17 mediate osteoclast formation through induction of RANKL [6]. Lymphocyte subsets (Th2) produce cytokines that are anti-inflammatory, IL-4 and IL-10. These cytokines reduce osteoclastogenesis and the severity of bone loss [7].

Mediators Involved in Bone Resorption

Mediators play an important role in the pathogenesis of bone damage. Cytokines stimulate the recruitment, formation and activity of the bone-resorbing cell, the osteoclast. They trigger the chemotaxis of osteoclast precursors, the induction of genes that lead to fusion of these precursors, the maturation of osteoclasts and the synthesis of matrix enzymes leading to bone resorption. Understanding these steps has led to the development of therapeutic agents that can block these osteoclastogenesis and activity reducing bone loss [8].

RANKL and CSF-1 work cooperatively and represent one of the dominant pathways that leads to osteoclast formation and activity [9]. CSF-1 is crucial for the proliferation and survival of osteoclast precursor cells, while RANKL is essential for osteoclast differentiation [9]. RANKL, also called tumor necrosis factor ligand superfamily member 11 is a cytokine that belongs to the TNF family. RANKL is expressed on the surface of marrow stromal cells, monocytes, activated T and B cells, osteocytes and precursors of bone forming osteoblasts. RANKL may be cleaved and released in a soluble form by metalloproteinases. It should be noted that the cell type that expresses RANKL may depend upon the etiology of the bone resorption. For example, the cells that produce RANKL differ between bone resorption caused by post-menopausal osteoporosis versus resorption associated with periodontal disease. During physiologic bone resorption, these factors act on osteoblasts/osteocytes to regulate RANKL and osteoprotegerin (OPG) expression.

CSF-1 also known as macrophage colony-stimulating factor (M-CSF) is a glycoprotein growth factor that specifically regulates the survival, proliferation and differentiation of monocyte-macrophage lineage cells through a cell surface receptor selectively expressed on these cell types, c-fms. M-CSF is released by osteoblasts and bone marrow progenitor cells that upon binding to its receptor, c-fms on pre-osteoclasts, activates an intracellular cascade that leads to proliferation of precursors and survival of osteoclasts. RANKL stimulates osteoclastogenesis when it binds to receptor activator of nuclear factor-κB (RANK), which is located on osteoclast precursors to activate NF-κB and other signaling pathways. This binding promotes osteoclast formation, activation, and survival, thus inducing osteoclast activity and bone resorption (fig. 1).

OPG, also called tumor necrosis factor-receptor superfamily member 11B (TNFRSF11B) is a soluble cytokine receptor that belongs to the TNF family [10]. It is produced by osteoblasts, fibroblasts and many other cell types. OPG binds to RANKL preventing RANKL from binding to its cognate receptor, RANK. Thus, OPG is a natural decoy receptor (inhibitor) of RANKL [11]. The RANKL/OPG expression ratio to a large degree determines the degree of osteoclast formation and activity [4].

A number of pro-inflammatory cytokines stimulate bone resorption [4] (fig. 1). Most accomplish this by stimulating production of RANKL. Some, such as TNF-α can induce RANKL but also stimulate osteoclast formation directly, independently of RANKL (fig. 1). TNF-α is produced primarily by activated macrophages, but also by other cell types such as activated T cells, polymorphonuclear leukocytes, epithelial cells, endothelial cells, fibroblasts and bone-lining cells including osteoblasts. TNF-α upregulates c-fms (CSF-1 receptor) expression and activates osteoclasts by enhancing RANKL signaling mechanisms. TNF-α induces osteoclast precursors and marrow stromal cells to produce osteoclastogenic cytokines, such as IL-1, RANKL, and M-CSF. TNF also inhibits the bone-forming function of osteoblasts. Studies show that TNF-α inhibits the differentiation of new osteoblasts from precursor cells. The regulation of RUNX2 by TNF could diminish recruitment of osteoblast precursors into the pool of mature bone-forming cells [12].

IL-1, which is encoded by two separate genes, IL-1α and IL-1β, is a potent bone resorbing cytokine produced by various cell types such as monocytes, macrophages, polymorphonuclear leukocytes, fibroblasts (gingival and periodontal ligament), epithelial cells, endothelial cells and osteoblasts. Both isoforms of IL-1 stimulate production of other cytokines and prostaglandins and can induce RANKL expression as well as production of degradative enzymes. However, it does

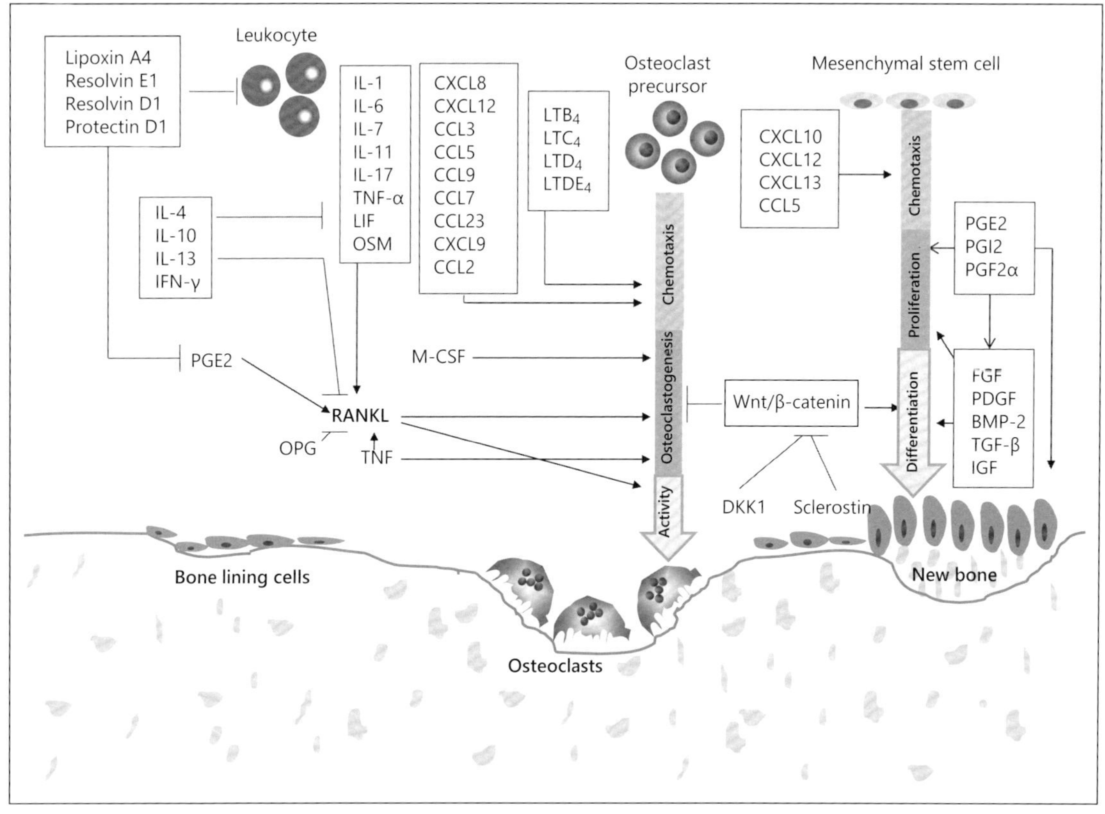

Fig. 1. Stimulation of osteoclastogenesis, bone resorption, and coupled bone formation. RANKL, M-CSF, and TNF directly stimulate the formation of osteoclasts, while other cytokines or lipid-based mediators such as prostaglandins or leukotrienes indirectly stimulate osteoclastogenesis by effects on RANKL, M-CSF, or TNF-α. Chemokines affect resorption by stimulation recruitment of osteoclast precursors or osteoclast activity. Chemokines such as CXCL10, CXCL12, CXCL13, and CCL5, may affect bone formation by effects on osteoblast precursors or osteoblasts. Wnt signaling, growth factors such as FGF, PDGF, BMP-2, TGF-β, and IGF play an important role in osteogenesis by stimulating proliferation of mesenchymal stem cells/osteoblast precursors and inducing osteoblast differentiation or synthesis of bone matrix. Modified with permission from Graves et al. [30].

not directly induce osteoclastogenesis [13]. IL-6 is produced by many of the same cell types that produce IL-1. IL-6 has been reported to stimulate bone resorption by enhancing osteoclast formation through a RANKL-dependent mechanism [14]. IL-7 is an osteoclastogenic cytokine mainly produced by stromal cells and osteoblasts that promotes RANKL expression. It also inhibits new bone formation by down regulation of the osteoblast-specific transcription factor Runx2. IL-17 is produced by activated CD4+ Th17 cells and stim-

ulates cells to express receptor activator of RANKL. IL-17 also reduces bone formation via inhibition of type I collagen synthesis [15]. Other osteoclastogenic cytokines that have been shown to stimulate activation of RANKL are IL-11, leukemia inhibitory factor, and oncostatin M (fig. 1).

Chemokines are chemotactic cytokines that stimulate recruitment of leukocytes and are produced by a wide variety of cell types including epithelial cells, endothelial cells, and many different leukocyte subsets of the innate and adaptive immune response, fibroblasts or bone lining cells [4]. Some chemokines recruit osteoclast precursors (fig. 1). CCL2 (also known as monocyte chemoattractant protein-1, MCP-1) induces recruitment of osteoclast precursors. Other chemokines that have been shown to stimulate recruitment of osteoclast precursors are CCL5, CXCL8, CCL9, CCL7, CCL23, CXCL12, and CXCL9 [4, 16, 17]. CCL3 (also called MIP-1α), a pro-inflammatory chemokine produced at inflammatory sites, appears to play a crucial role in pathologic osteoclastogenesis associated with multiple myelomas. It modulates osteoclast differentiation by binding to G-protein coupled receptors, CCR1 and CCR5, and activating ERK and AKT signaling pathways. The MIP-1β (CCL4) also can enhance bone resorption [16, 17].

Prostaglandins and leukotrienes are lipid-based mediators derived from fatty acids that are produced by different cell types such as macrophages, fibroblasts and gingival epithelial cells (fig. 1) [18]. Prostaglandin E (PGEs), such as prostaglandin E_2, prostacyclin and prostaglandin $F_{2\alpha}$ stimulate osteoclast formation through RANKL and direct effect on osteoclast formation, also stimulate bone formation. Prostaglandin E_2 has been linked to stimulating insulin growth factor-1 gene expression, which promotes collagen synthesis by osteoblasts, thus enhancing bone formation [19]. Leukotrienes are another class of inflammatory lipid mediators and stimulate chemotaxis of leukocytes and the generation of superoxides in neutrophils. Leukotrienes such as LTB_4, LTC_4, LTD_4 and $LTDE_4$ enhance osteoclast formation and activation of mature osteoclasts by a RANKL independent mechanism. LTB_4 may suppress bone formation by inhibiting the proliferation of primary osteoblast precursors and reduce the capacity of osteoblast precursors to differentiate into osteoblasts and form new bone [20]. Lipoxins and the D and E series of resolvins are endogenous anti-inflammatory lipid mediators that act by controlling the resolution of the inflammation through enhancing apoptosis of

PMNs and their clearance by macrophages, blocking leukotrienes and prostaglandins as well as reducing cytokine release [21]. For example, resolvin E1 is produced during the resolution of the inflammation and blocks stimulation by leukotriene B4. This inhibition attenuates neutrophil migration leading thereby reducing inflammation. Lipoxin acts by binding to lipoxin A4 receptor inhibiting chemotaxis, transmigration and blocking activation of nuclear factor kappa-B.

Matrix metalloproteinases (MMPs) are proteases produced by different cell types such as macrophages and fibroblasts [22]. Inflammatory mediators induce production of MMP from a number of cell types such as fibroblasts and PMNs. These molecules degrade extracellular matrix proteins such as collagen, elastin, and laminins. Osteoclasts secrete MMP contributing to degradation of bone matrix following decalcification by acid production. Furthermore, MMPs can activate chemokines and cytokines to amplify inflammation [23]. For example, MMPs activate chemokines by cleavage of the N-terminal domain.

Mediators That Stimulate Bone Formation

Wnt signaling, growth factors and bone morphogenetic proteins play an important role in osteogenesis [24, 27, 28] (fig. 1). The Wnt signaling transduction pathway plays an important role in stimulating bone formation and in many other processes including embryonic development and tumorigenesis [24]. Wnts are secreted, cysteine-rich glycoproteins involved in controlling cell proliferation, cell-fate specification, gene expression, and cell survival. Wnt-3a and Wnt-7a are expressed in the limb bud and have roles in skeletal pattern determination, while Wnt-14 is involved in joint formation. And Wnt-3a, Wnt-4, Wnt-5a, and Wnt-7a all influence cartilage development. Wnt receptors are including low-density lipoprotein receptor-related proteins (LRP) and frizzleds

(Fzd). LRP are evolutionarily conserved plasma membrane receptors with a variety of functions including lipid metabolism, cargo transport, and cellular signaling. LRP-5 is expressed by osteoblasts of the endosteal and trabecular bone surface. It regulates osteoblastic proliferation, survival and activity. Fzds are highly versatile seven-membrane proteins that contribute to activation of both β-catenin and non-β-catenin signaling pathways by virtue of their interactions with Dishevelled (Dsh, or Dvl), a cytoplasmic phosphoprotein that acts directly downstream of frizzled receptors. The Wnt pathway has been found to play a central role in controlling embryonic bone development and bone mass. There are four Wnt pathways: the canonical Wnt pathway (the Wnt/b-catenin pathway) and three non-canonical Wnt (β-catenin independent) pathways: the Wnt/Ca2þ pathway, the Wnt/planar cell polarity (Wnt/PCP) pathway, and the Wnt/protein kinase A (Wnt/PKA) pathway. Beta-catenin, a key component of the canonical Wnt signaling pathway interacts with a number of different transcription factors and modulates their activity. This leads to the transcription of a number of different target genes that regulate a diverse array of biological processes. In the osteocyte Wnt/beta-catenin signaling is required for normal bone homeostasis [24]. The Wnt/beta-catenin pathway is anabolic for bone formation and promotes increased bone density and strength. Beta-catenin activation facilitates osteoblast differentiation and enhances osteoblast and osteocyte survival in vitro. The Wnt pathway can also affect osteoclastogenesis. The Wnt/beta-catenin pathway suppresses physiologic bone resorption by upregulation of OPG expression and downregulation of RANKL in osteoblasts/osteocytes [25].

The Wnt pathway is inhibited by Dickkopf factors 1–4 (DKK1, DKK2, DKK3, DKK4) and sclerostin. Dkk1 is expressed by synovial cells, endothelial cells and chondrocytes. Dickkopf factors, especially DKK1, bind and sequester the LRP5/6 and Kremen1/2 (Krm1/2), the Wnt pathway receptors membrane complex to inhibit Wnt activity. Sclerostin, the protein product of the Sost gene is also a Wnt inhibitor. It is produced by osteocytes and is abundant in osteocytic canaliculae. Sclerostin binds to Lrp5/6 to block the Wnt/beta-catenin pathway and inhibit proliferation and differentiation of osteoblasts and to increase their apoptosis [25].

Fibroblast growth factor-2 (FGF-2 also known as basic FGF) is involved in numerous cellular processes including angiogenesis, tumorigenesis, cell proliferation, differentiation, wound healing, limb formation, and bone biology. In bone, FGF-2 is expressed in osteoblasts and mesenchymal cells. Postnatally, FGF-2 is produced by mature osteoblasts and stored in extracellular matrix. FGF-2 along with FGF-18 is a bone anabolic agent that stimulates uncommitted bone marrow stromal cells to differentiate into osteoblasts and form osteoid. Thus it plays an important role in skeletal development by regulating the proliferation and differentiation of osteoblasts [26]. FGF-2 signaling regulates the Wnt/beta-catenin pathway and activates transcription factors Runx2 and activating transcription factor 4 (ATF4), thereby promoting osteoblast differentiation [27].

Bone morphogenetic proteins (BMPs) are a group of protein factors that stimulate bone formation and are important in a number of other biologic factors such as skin formation and hair follicle development [28] (fig. 1). BMPs released by osteoclasts and from resorbing bone matrix interact with specific receptors on the cell surface, referred to as bone morphogenetic protein receptors (BMPRs). There are type I and type II BMPRs. Two subclasses of type I receptors have been identified, type IA and IB (BMPR1A and BMPR1B). Upon ligand binding, the type II receptor forms a heterodimer with the type I receptor, and the constitutive kinase of the type II activates the type I receptor. The latter initiates a signal transduction cascade by phosphorylating downstream cytosolic factors, which then translocate to the nucleus to activate or inhibit transcription. Signaling by BMPs plays an important role in variety of cell types in bone such as osteoblasts and chondrocytes. BMPs have widely recognized roles in bone formation such as BMP-2, BMP-4, BMP-5, BMP-6 and BMP-7 which have an osteogenic capacity. BMPs stimulate intracellular signaling by activating the mothers against decapentaplegic (Smad) and mitogen-activated protein kinase (MAPK) pathways. Following BMP induction, both the Smad and MAPK pathways converge at the Runx2 gene to control its activation. The subsequent signaling induced by BMP (ligand, receptors, intracellular mediators, activation of transcription factors or comodulators) is responsible for the final target gene expression. BMP signaling may also be required for expression of RANKL in osteoblasts/osteocytes [28]. BMP signaling can be inhibited or modified in many ways, including inhibition through chordin and noggin. These antagonists are regulated by BMPs, indicating the existence of local feedback mechanisms to modulate BMP cellular activities. For example, noggin binds with various degrees of affinity to BMP-2, BMP-4, BMP-5, BMP-6 and BMP-7. Crystallography of noggin and BMP-7 reveals that noggin inhibits BMP-7 signaling by blocking the molecular interfaces of the binding epitopes for both type I and type II BMP receptors. Basal noggin expression in osteoblasts is limited but its transcript levels are upregulated by BMP-2, BMP-4 and BMP-6 as a potential protective mechanism limiting excessive BMP stimulation [29].

References

1 Schett G, Teitelbaum SL: Osteoclasts and arthritis. J Bone Miner Res 2009;24: 1142–1146.

2 Jiao H, Xiao E, Graves DT: Diabetes and its effect on bone and fracture healing. Curr Osteoporos Rep 2015;13:327–335.

3 Karsenty G: Transcriptional control of skeletogenesis. Annu Rev Genomics Hum Genet 2008;9:183–196.

4 Graves DT, Oates T, Garlet GP: Review of osteoimmunology and the host response in endodontic and periodontal lesions. J Oral Microbiol 2011;3:10.3402.

5 Benoit M, Desnues B, Mege JL: Macrophage polarization in bacterial infections. J Immunol 2008;181:3733–3739.

6 Sato K, Suematsu A, Okamoto K, et al: Th17 functions as an osteoclastogenic helper T cell subset that links T cell activation and bone destruction. J Exp Med 2006;203:2673–2682.

7 Dinarello CA: Historical insights into cytokines. Eur J Immunol 2007;37(suppl 1):S34–S45.

8 Schett G: Effects of inflammatory and anti-inflammatory cytokines on the bone. Eur J Clin Invest 2011;41:1361–1366.

9 Takayanagi H: Osteoimmunology: shared mechanisms and crosstalk between the immune and bone systems. Nat Rev Immunol 2007;7:292–304.

10 Belibasakis GN, Bostanci N: The RANKL-OPG system in clinical periodontology. J Clin Periodontol 2012;39: 239–248.

11 Simonet WS, Lacey DL, Dunstan CR, et al: Osteoprotegerin: a novel secreted protein involved in the regulation of bone density. Cell 1997;89:309–319.

12 Karmakar S, Kay J, Gravallese EM: Bone damage in rheumatoid arthritis: mechanistic insights and approaches to prevention. Rheum Dis Clin North Am 2010;36:385–404.

13 Nagai H, Tsukuda R, Mayahara H: Effects of basic fibroblast growth factor (bFGF) on bone formation in growing rats. Bone 1995;16:367–373.

14 Palmqvist P, Persson E, Conaway HH, Lerner UH: IL-6, leukemia inhibitory factor, and oncostatin M stimulate bone resorption and regulate the expression of receptor activator of NF-kappa B ligand, osteoprotegerin, and receptor activator of NF-kappa B in mouse calvariae. J Immunol 2002;169:3353–3362.

15 Daoussis D, Andonopoulos AP, Liossis SN: Wnt pathway and IL-17:novel regulators of joint remodeling in rheumatic diseases. Looking beyond the RANK-RANKL-OPG axis. Semin Arthritis Rheum 2010;39:369–383.

16 Szekanecz Z, Koch AE, Tak PP: Chemokine and chemokine receptor blockade in arthritis, a prototype of immune-mediated inflammatory diseases. Neth J Med 2011;69:356–366.

17 Szekanecz Z, Vegvari A, Szabo Z, Koch AE: Chemokines and chemokine receptors in arthritis. Front Biosci (Schol Ed) 2010;2:153–167.

18 Bage T, Kats A, Lopez BS, et al: Expression of prostaglandin E synthases in periodontitis immunolocalization and cellular regulation. Am J Pathol 2011; 178:1676–1688.

19 Minamizaki T, Yoshiko Y, Kozai K, Aubin JE, Maeda N: EP2 and EP4 receptors differentially mediate MAPK pathways underlying anabolic actions of prostaglandin E2 on bone formation in rat calvaria cell cultures. Bone 2009;44: 1177–1185.

20 Jiang J, Lv HS, Lin JH, Jiang DF, Chen ZK: LTB4 can directly stimulate human osteoclast formation from PBMC independent of RANKL. Artif Cells Blood Substit Immobil Biotechnol 2005;33: 391–403.

21 Serhan CN, Chiang N, Van Dyke TE: Resolving inflammation: dual anti-inflammatory and pro-resolution lipid mediators. Nat Rev Immunol 2008;8: 349–361.

22 Manicone AM, McGuire JK: Matrix metalloproteinases as modulators of inflammation. Semin Cell Dev Biol 2008; 19:34–41.

23 Giannobile WV: Host-response therapeutics for periodontal diseases. J Periodontol 2008;79:1592–1600.

24 Chen Y, Alman BA: Wnt pathway, an essential role in bone regeneration. J Cell Biochem 2009;106:353–362.

25 Takahashi N, Maeda K, Ishihara A, Uehara S, Kobayashi Y: Regulatory mechanism of osteoclastogenesis by RANKL and Wnt signals. Front Biosci 2011;16: 21–30.

26 Downey ME, Holliday LS, Aguirre JI, Wronski TJ: In vitro and in vivo evidence for stimulation of bone resorption by an EP4 receptor agonist and basic fibroblast growth factor: Implications for their efficacy as bone anabolic agents. Bone 2009;44:266–274.

27 Ai-Aql ZS, Alagl AS, Graves DT, Gerstenfeld LC, Einhorn TA: Molecular mechanisms controlling bone formation during fracture healing and distraction osteogenesis. J Dent Res 2008;87:107–118.

28 Chen G, Deng C, Li YP: TGF-beta and BMP signaling in osteoblast differentiation and bone formation. Int J Biol Sci 2012;8:272–288.

29 Krause C, Guzman A, Knaus P· Noggin. Int J Biochem Cell Biol 2011;43:478–481.

30 Graves DT, Li J, Cochran DL: Inflammation and uncoupling as mechanisms of periodontal bone loss. J Dent Res 2011; 90:143–153.

Dana Graves
Department of Periodontics, University of Pennsylvania
240 S. 40th St., Levy 122
Philadelphia, PA 19104 (USA)
E-Mail dtgraves@dental.upenn.edu

Kantarci A, Will L, Yen S (eds): Tooth Movement. Front Oral Biol. Basel, Karger, 2016, vol 18, pp 17–27
DOI: 10.1159/000351896

Bone Remodeling Under Pathological Conditions

Wenmei Xiao[a, d] · Shuai Li[b, d] · Sandra Pacios[d, e] · Yu Wang[c, d] · Dana T. Graves[d]

Departments of [a]Periodontology and [b]Implantology, School and Hospital of Stomatology, Peking University, Beijing, and [c]Department of Dental Implantology, School and Hospital of Stomatology, Jilin University, Jilin, PR China; [d]Department of Periodontics, School of Dental Medicine, University of Pennsylvania, Philadelphia, Pa., USA; [e]Department of Periodontology, School of Dental Medicine, Universitat Internacional de Catalunya, Sant Cugat del Vallès, Spain

Abstract

Bone is masterfully programmed to repair itself through the coupling of bone formation following bone resorption, a process referred to as coupling. In inflammatory or other conditions, the balance between bone resorption and bone formation shifts so that a net bone loss results. This review focuses on four pathologic conditions in which remodeling leads to net loss of bone, postmenopausal osteoporosis, arthritis, periodontal disease, and disuse bone loss, which is similar to bone loss associated with microgravity. In most of these there is an acceleration of the resorptive process due to increased formation of bone metabolic units. This initially leads to a net bone loss since the time period of resorption is much faster than the time needed for bone formation that follows. In addition, each of these processes is characterized by an uncoupling that leads to net bone loss. Mechanisms responsible for increased rates of bone resorption, i.e. the formation of more bone metabolic units, involve enhanced expression of inflammatory cytokines and increased expression of RANKL. Moreover, the reasons for uncoupling are discussed which range from a decrease in expression of growth factors and bone morphogenetic proteins to increased expression of factors that inhibit Wnt signaling.   © 2016 S. Karger AG, Basel

Bone Remodeling in Postmenopausal Osteoporosis

Osteoporosis is one of the most common metabolic bone diseases and a leading cause of morbidity in our aging population [1]. The most common form of osteoporosis in women is postmenopausal osteoporosis, which is also called primary type 1 osteoporosis. Primary type 2 osteoporosis occurs in the elderly in both females and males and is due to aging. In addition, osteoporosis may occur for other reasons such as long term use of glucocorticoids, which is referred to as secondary osteoporosis. Increased risk of fracture and pain due to spinal compression caused by osteoporosis are the most significant morbid consequences of osteoporosis. Trabecular bone undergoes more extensive remodeling than cortical bone. As a result osteoporosis has a greater effect on trabecular than cortical bone. A characteristic feature of osteoporosis is a disrupted micro architecture of trabecular bone with reduced and weaker trabecular spicules. Common sites of osteoporosis involve the wrist, the hip and the spine, which have relatively large ratios of trabecular to cortical bone.

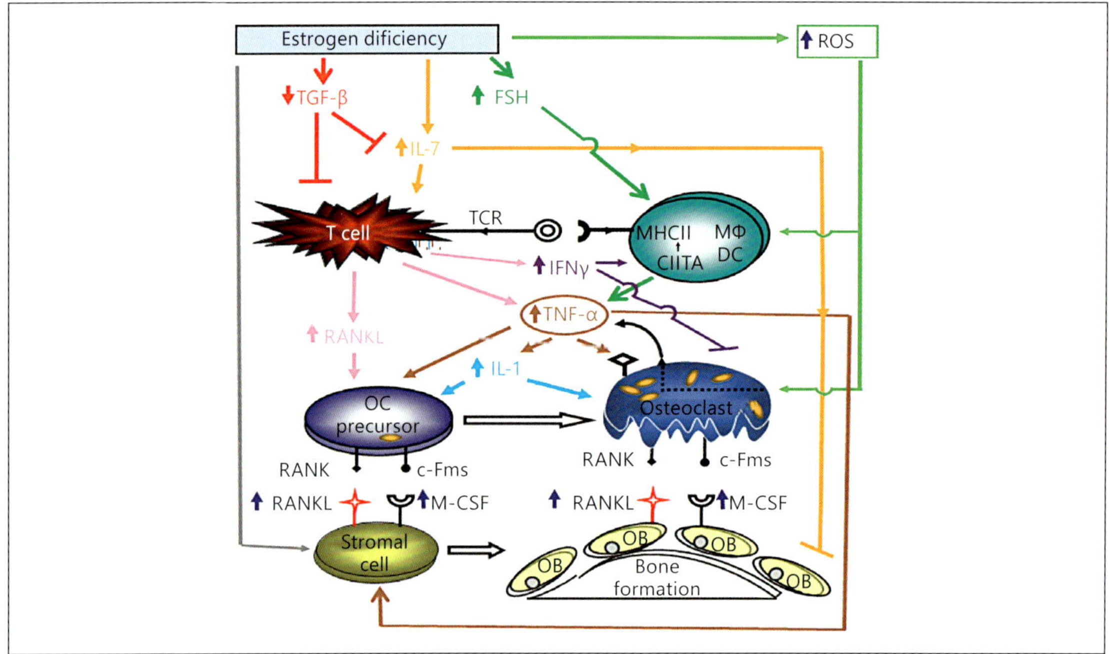

Fig. 1. Schematic representation of the main mechanisms and feedback interactions by which estrogen deficiency leads to bone loss. The bone loss induced by estrogen deficiency is caused, in part by the increase in FSH which results from estrogen deficiency. Estrogen deficiency leads to a global increase in IL-7 production in target organs such as bone, in part through decreases in TGF-β. This leads to a first wave of T cell activation. Activated T cells release IFN-γ, which increase Ag presentation by dendritic cells and macrophages by upregulating MHCII expression through the transcription factor CIITA. Estrogen deficiency also amplifies T cell activation and osteoclastogenesis by downregulating antioxidant pathways leading to an upswing in ROS. The resulting increase in ROS stimulates Ag presentation and the production of TNF by mature osteoclasts. The combined effect of IFNγ and ROS markedly enhances Ag presentation, amplifying T cell activation and promoting release of the osteoclastogenic factors TNF and RANKL. TNF further stimulates stromal cell and osteoblast RANKL and macrophage colony-stimulating factor production further driving up osteoclast formation. TNF stimulates the production of IL-1 which influences osteoclast formation and activity. IL-7 further exacerbates bone loss by blunting bone formation through direct repressive effects on osteoblasts. From Pacifici [2], reprinted with permission.

Postmenopausal osteoporosis is associated with decreased gonadal function. Both a decreased of estrogen and an increased in follicle-stimulating hormone (FSH) production secondary to estrogen deficiency contribute to postmenopausal bone loss [1, 2] (fig. 1). Estrogens are produced primarily by developing follicles in the ovaries. Estrogens inhibit formation of bone metabolic units (BMUs) by decreasing the production of osteoclast-activating cytokines such as IL-1, IL-6, IL-7 and tumor necrosis factor-α (TNF-α) and by promoting osteoclast apoptosis. In addition, estrogens increase the production of OPG which opposes bone resorption. Likewise, estrogens promote bone formation by increasing the production of insulin-like growth factor-1 and transforming growth factor (TGF) [2]. In healthy young adults, bone resorption and bone formation are in balance, a process called coupling. Coupling results from the formation of BMU, a temporary anatomical structure that forms a bone-remodeling compartment. An active BMU consists of a leading front of bone resorbing osteoclasts, reversal cells covering the newly exposed bone surface prepare it for osteoblasts. Osteoblasts then occupy the trailing portion of the BMU and secrete and deposit unmineralized bone matrix known as osteoid. In humans osteoclasts require weeks to resorb bone and osteoblasts require months to produce new bone. Thus, processes that increase the rate of bone remodeling initially results in net bone loss, i.e. resorption initially exceeds formation since formation takes a much longer period of time even if coupling is normal.

The primary causes of postmenopausal osteoporosis both of which are linked to estrogen deficiency are increased bone resorption and decreased bone formation. Estrogen deficiency is associated with increased formation of discrete resorptive foci on the endosteal surfaces of bone. The increased number of remodeling events and the reduced formation of bone from each BMU results in relatively rapid loss of trabecular bone after menopause. Other cellular events that are enhanced in postmenopausal osteoporosis include recruitment of osteoclasts precursors to the bone surfaces and an increase in the lifespan of osteoclasts. Osteoblast expression of OPG is decreased after menopause and production of CSF-1 and RANKL by osteoblast and stromal cell is increased to promote proliferation of osteoclast precursors and differentiation of mature osteoclasts (fig. 1). Due to estrogen deficiency and an increase in FSH there is an increase in the number of TNF-producing T cells. The activation of T cells can be also enhanced by estrogen deficiency through upregulating of interferon-γ (IFN-γ) and reactive oxygen species (ROS), which markedly enhances antigen (Ag) presentation by dendritic cells and macrophages. Thus, activated T cells enhance RANKL-induced osteoclast formation and bone loss. Estrogen deficiency also upregulates inflammatory cytokine production as mentioned above, such as IL-7 and TNF, which not only enhance osteoclastogenesis also limit functional activating of mature osteoblasts [2]. It is reported that due to estrogen deficiency there is increased activation of nuclear factor-κ B in osteoblasts that inhibit its function, limiting the bone formation and contributing to uncoupling of bone formation and resorption [3]. The increase in nuclear factor-κ B is thought to cause uncoupling because it decreases expression of Fra-1, which is needed to optimally produce bone matrix.

In summary, it is a complex pathway associated with estrogen and the immune system by which estrogen deficiency leads to bone loss after postmenopausal osteoporosis. Estrogen deficiency induces T cell activation in part by stimulating Ag presentation, and in part via stimulation of IL-7 production and through decreases in transforming growth factor-β (TGF-β). Estrogen deficiency also amplifies T cell activation by downregulating antioxidant pathways leading to increases in ROS. Activated T cells release the osteoclastogenic factors TNF and RANKL, which result in osteoclasts formation and bone loss (fig. 1).

Because postmenopausal osteoporosis involves both increased bone resorption and decreased bone coupling, both aspects of bone remodeling can be therapeutically targeted [1, 4]. Antiresorptive treatments include the use of bisphosphonate, which decreases bone resorption by blocking farnesyl-diphosphate synthase and inhibiting the HMG CoA-reductase pathway. This decreases the formation of osteoclasts as well as increases osteoclast apoptosis. Although statins have a similar effect in blocking the HMG CoA-reductase pathway, statins do not bind to bone and as a result are not thought to be as useful in treating osteoporosis. Estrogen replacement therapy is effective in treating osteoporosis because it reverses the loss of estrogen which is a primary trigger in post-menopausal osteoporosis. However, due to risks of treatment with estrogen it is not as commonly used. Selective estrogen receptor modulators bind to subclasses of estrogen receptors and do not have the disadvantages of estrogen treatment. An example of a selective estrogen receptor modulator is raloxifene.

Calcitonin, given by nasal spray is another treatment of osteoporosis that inhibits cytoskeletal function in osteoclasts thereby inhibiting osteoclast function. Denosumab is a humanized monoclonal antibody that binds to RANKL and inhibits it thereby blocking formation of osteoclasts. The primary anabolic treatment of osteoporosis is through teriparatide, a recombinant peptide (1–34 amino acids) of parathyroid hormone that is injected once daily. Although teriparatide stimulates bone resorption intermittent exposure has a greater effect on osteoblasts than osteoclasts leading to a net increase in bone formation.

Bone Remodeling in Arthritis

Rheumatoid arthritis (RA) is a chronic and progressive systemic inflammatory disease characterized by particular inflammation leading to erosion of joint pain and loss of cartilage [5–7]. Approximately 1% of the population has RA, which is much more common in women than men. Like periodontal disease, onset often occurs between the ages of 40 and 50. A characteristic feature is synovitis which is inflammation of the synovial membrane that lines joints. Inflammation of the joints caused by RA is painful and can lead to loss of function. Lymphocytes play a key role in RA. There may be a genetic linkage to disease susceptibility and it appears that RA is aggravated by smoking. There is significant improvement in RA by inhibition of TNF or a depletion of B lymphocytes demonstrating the importance of TNF and B cells in the disease progression. Data from clinical trials confirm that depleting B cells slows progression of bone loss and erosion of joint cartilage space narrowing. This finding supports a significant role for B cells in the pathogenesis of bone and joint destruction in RA [5]. In addition, auto antibodies are present as well as antibodies to citrullinated peptides. It has been suggested that RA involves abnormal B cell-T cell interactions in which B cells present antigen to T cells. The formation of immune complexes may aggravate the disease. It is possible that the etiology that imitates autoimmunity may be distinguished from the inflammation that drives the debilitating disease process.

RA causes resorption of subchondral bone and can lead to a more systemic bone loss [5–8] (fig. 2). RA is the most common systemic autoimmune disease. The hyperinflammatory response in RA involves dysregulation of both adaptive and innate immunity. Cells of the innate immune response that have been shown to participate in RA include PMNs, monocytes/macrophages and dendritic cells. PMNs increase bone resorption by activating monocyte fusion into fully functional osteoclasts. In addition to recruitment of monocytes there is also local proliferation of macrophages in areas of inflammation in RA. Increased macrophage activation in RA results in the expression of chemokines, such as CXCL-12 (SDF-1), CCL3 (MIP-1α) and CCL20 that attract leukocytes to areas of inflammation [8]. There is a correlation between synovial macrophage infiltration and subsequent radiographic joint destruction. Dendritic cells have a role in osteolysis in RA through the activation of Th17 cells by producing IL-6, TGF-β and IL-23, which then can stimulate osteoclast differentiation and bone resorption by expressing RANKL (fig. 2). In addition, lymphocytes produce factors such as IFN-γ that enhance activity of the innate immune response further increasing inflammation and the production of bone-resorptive cytokines. Th1 and Th17 cells have been implicated in RA. Th1 and Th2 cells inhibit osteoclastogenesis through the production of IFN-γ and IL-4, respectively, but its overall affect in vivo is to increase osteoclastogenesis because it stimulates inflammatory responses in other cell types. Th17 cells promote bone loss in RA by producing IL-17 [6].

One hypothesis for RA is that there is a cytokine imbalance caused by skewing of lymphocyte differentiation that favors Th1 and Th17 cells at the expense of Th2 and T regulatory lymphocytes. This skewing can lead to over production of

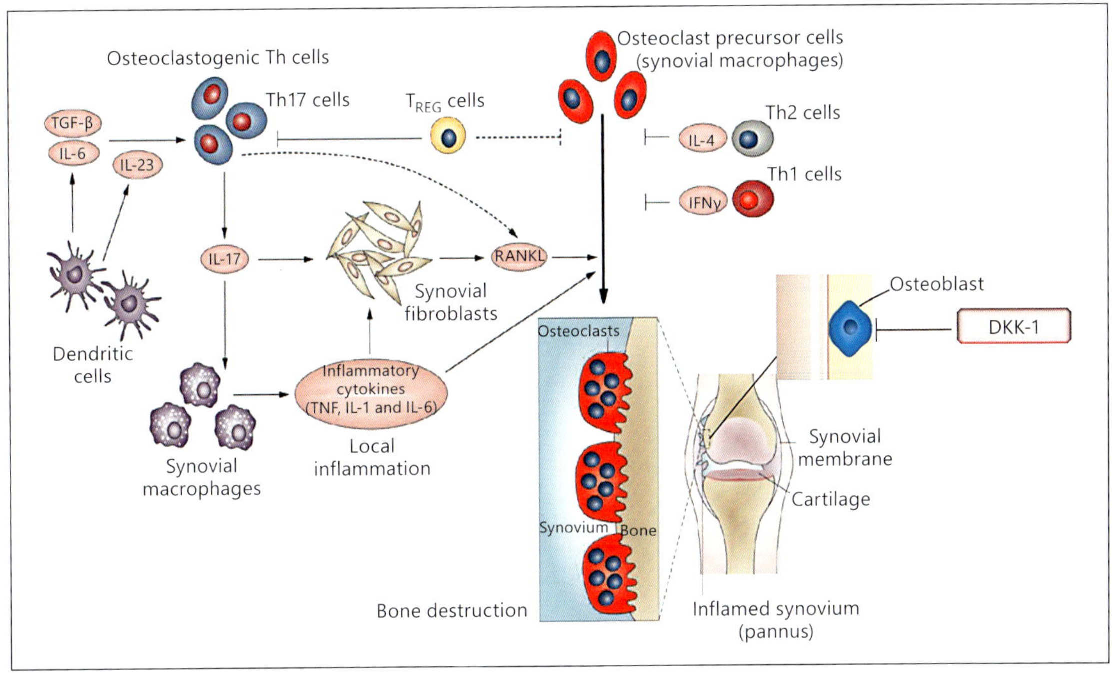

Fig. 2. In the pathogenesis of bone destruction associated with RA, the immune cells play an important role. Th17 cells secrete a huge amount of IL-17, which induces RANKL on synovial fibroblasts and stimulates local inflammation and activates synovial macrophages to secrete proinflammatory cytokines, such as TNF, IL-1 and IL-6. The induction of Th17 cells is regulated by IL-6, TGF- and IL-23 produced by dendritic cells. Th1 and Th2 cells inhibit osteoclastogenesis through the production of IFN-γ and IL-4, respectively. Joint remodeling in RA is driven by RANKL-mediated osteoclast activation and bone resorption, which form bone erosions. At the same time, DKK-1, a Wnt inhibitor, blocks bone formation by inhibiting osteoblasts. From Takayanagi et al. [28], reprinted with permission.

TNF-α, IL-1, IL-6, IL-13, IL-15, IL-17, IL-18 and IL-22. TNF-α is an important mediator in the pathogenesis of RA and has received considerable attention because of its position as an early mediator in the pro-inflammatory cytokine cascade [6]. It is synthesized primarily by macrophages and synovial lining cells, as well as by activated T cells. It is reported that TNF-α can increase the number of osteoclast precursor cells in vivo. Blocking TNF-α reduces osteoclastogenesis and bone resorption in RA. Data from clinical trials confirm that inhibiting TNF-α activity in RA effectively protects against bone erosion [7]. TNF-α can increases the rate of synthesis of metalloproteinases by synovial macrophages and fibroblasts, and inhibit the synthesis of proteoglycans in car-

tilage. Inhibition of TNF-α can also reduce clinical signs and symptoms of disease [7].

Other prominent pro-inflammatory cytokines that are involved in RA include IL-1, IL-6 and IL-17 [6]. High levels of IL-1, IL-6 and IL-17 have been detected in synovial fluid specimens obtained from patients with RA. These pro-inflammatory mediators induce bone resorption associated with RA largely through stimulation of RANKL. In vivo studies indicate that these mediators contribute to bone loss in RA. Over-expression of IL-1 or deficiency of the soluble IL-1 receptor antagonist results in greater bone destruction in animal models of RA. Administration of blocking antibodies against the IL-6 receptor significantly reduced osteoclast formation and bone erosion in vivo. Blocking IL-17 in vivo reduces joint inflammation and bone erosion by suppressing RANKL, IL-1, and TNF-α production [5].

Chemokines take part in the process of the bone destruction in RA [8]. They are abundantly expressed in the sera, synovial fluids and tissues of arthritis patients. They induce recruitment of osteoclast precursors and have been reported stimulate some steps in osteoclastogenesis [8]. They can also indirectly participate in osteoclastogenesis by stimulating the recruitment of inflammatory cells, which in turn induce or express TNF-α or RANKL. For example, CCL20 recruits Th17 cells that express IL-17 but also has the capacity to directly affect osteoclastogenesis by increasing the number of preosteoclasts [8].

RANKL is an important osteoclastogenic factor present within the RA synovium and it is the product of synovial fibroblasts, T cells and macrophages [5, 6]. In RANKL-deficient mice bone destruction is blocked in an arthritis model but other destructive events involving cartilage erosion still occur [5, 6]. Consistent with this, anti-RANKL and anti-osteoclast therapies have been shown to be beneficial in the treatment of bone damage in animal models of RA [5, 6].

An important component of bone loss in RA is due to uncoupling. It is reported that in patients with RA, that Wnt signaling is blocked which contributes to uncoupling by interfering with bone formation. Thus, decreased Wnt signaling may be one mechanism by which osteoblast-mediated bone formation is compromised at sites of focal bone erosion in RA. Recent evidence suggests that this inhibition is due to increased expression of DKK-1 that is stimulated by high levels of TNF. Blockade of DKK-1 prevents net bone loss from restoring coupling after bone resorption and rescues the inhibition of osteoblastogenesis in RA [7].

In summary, the pathogenesis of RA bone destruction is associated with immune system and inflammatory cytokines, in which immune cells play an important role. Th17 cells regulated by cytokines produced from dendritic cells, such as IL-6, TGF-β and IL-23. Th17 cells secrete a huge amount of IL-17, which is associated with other pro-inflammatory cytokines to induce bone resorption through stimulation of RANKL (fig. 2).

Bone Remodeling in Periodontal Disease

Periodontal disease is a chronic inflammatory disease initiated by bacterial plaque that lead to a loss of connective tissue attachment and bone [9]. It is the most prevalent of the lytic bone disorder in humans and when severe can lead to tooth loss as demonstrated in 8–9% of adults in the United States [9–11]. There are over 700 bacterial species in the mouth. A relatively small portion of these are thought to initiate periodontal disease. Bacteria colonize the tooth surface and they or their products penetrate into the connective tissue to stimulate an inflammatory response [9–11]. The inflammatory response rather than the direct pathologic effects of the bacteria are thought to cause the tissue destruction of periodontal disease.

Leukocytes play an important role in periodontal disease [9, 10] (fig. 3). It is too simplistic to say that a particular leukocyte subset is protective or destructive since in protecting the host against bacterial challenge they elaborate factors that locally cause destruction. For example, PMNs produce oxygen radicals, proinflammatory lipid mediators such as leukotrienes and inflammatory cytokines such as TNF-α that contribute to the antibacterial defense but also contribute to tissue injury [11]. Macrophages similarly play a role in both by participating in anti-bacterial defense (phagocytosis and antigen-presenting cells) and removal of cellular debris. But they also contribute to inflammation and tissue loss. Dendritic cells (DCs) regulate inflammation by activating lymphocytes. Moreover, DCs may also act as osteoclast precursors that can develop into DC-derived osteoclasts under inflammatory conditions. Other cells that are also important in the fight

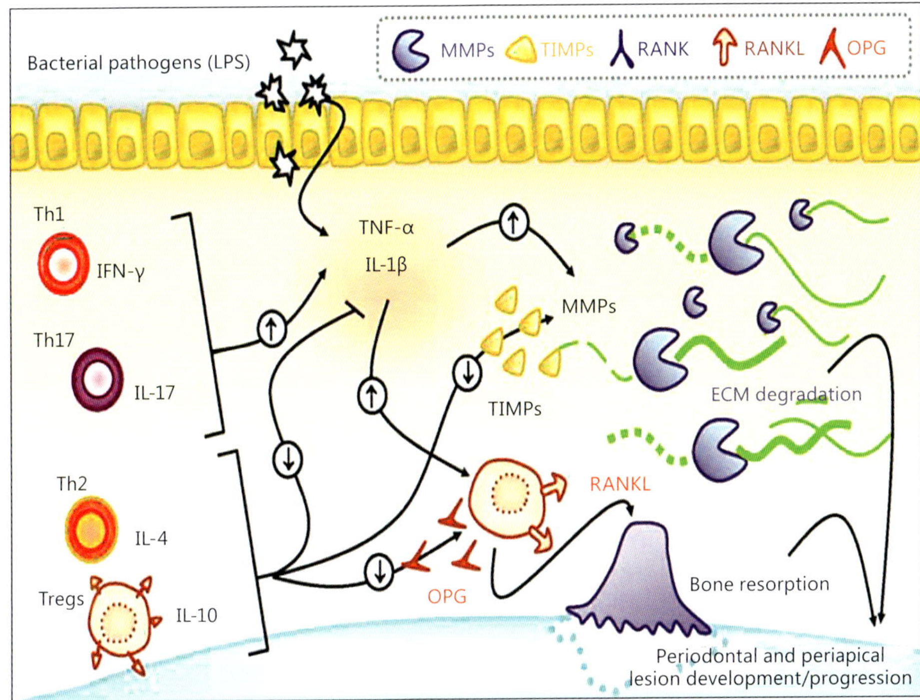

Fig. 3. Cytokine regulation of matrix degradation and bone resorption in periodontal and periapical environments. The presence of microbial pathogens in periodontal and periapical environments trigger an initial production of proinflammatory cytokines, such as TNF-α and IL-1β, which stimulate expression and activation of matrix metalloproteinases that degrade extracellular connective tissue matrix. Cytokines such as TNF-α can stimulate osteoclastogenesis independently while other cytokines stimulate RANKL expression that leads to formation of osteoclasts and osteoclast activity. The combined innate and adaptive immune responses are likely to lead to the high levels of inflammation and bone resorption. These proinflammatory cytokines are thought to generate an amplification loop that contributes to periodontal and periapical lesion progression. Conversely, cytokines produced by Th2 cells and Tregs, such as IL-4 and IL-10 have the opposite effect, in part, through stimulating production of tissue inhibitors of matrix metalloproteinases and OPG as well as restrain inflammatory cytokine production. From Graves et al. [10], reprinted with permission.

against bacteria are B and T cells. High levels of B cells are found when there is persistence of an inflammatory infiltrate. They can express RANKL causing periodontal bone loss. B cells differentiate to plasma cells that produce a variety of immunoglobulin enhancing the inflammatory response [10, 12]. T cells are also found in the dense inflammatory infiltrate of the periodontal disease and are found in various subtypes including naïve, memory, T regulatory, CD8+ and various CD4+ T helper cells (Th1, Th2 and Th17).

Inflammatory mediators are upregulated in periodontal disease [9, 10]. A number of studies have shown that inhibition of prostaglandins, IL-1, TNF, IL-6 and IFN-γ reduce periodontal inflammation and periodontal bone loss. Chemokines are also highly involved in periodontal disease. It is possible that chemokines, in addition to the classical cytokines, are involved in the immunopathogenesis of periodontal disease. They stimulate the migration and the maintenance of several inflammatory cell types such as polymorphonuclear leukocytes, DCs, natural killer cells, macrophages, and subsets of lymphocytes in the gingival tissues. Moreover, chemokines can act as chemoattractants for osteoclast precursors and activators of osteoclastogenesis [13]. RANKL and OPG can be detected in gingival tissue and biological fluids, including gingival crevicular fluid. RANKL is increased whereas OPG is decreased in periodontitis compared to health, or gingivitis [9, 10, 13]. It is produced as a membrane-bound or secreted ligand primarily by T cells, B cells and monocytes in periodontitis as well as minor production by other cell types. Inhibition of RANKL by antibody or OPG causes a decrease in alveolar bone loss in different models of periodontal disease [14].

Various cytokines produced during periodontal disease may also affect bone formation by modulating osteoblasts like IL-1 and IL-6, TNF-α, leukotrienes and matrix metalloproteinases [9, 10] (fig. 3). Matrix metalloproteinase upregulation has been seen to impede osteoblast differentiation of osteogenic PDL cells and consequently diminish bone regeneration [15]. Thus, high levels in periodontal disease are linked to decreased bone formation that is reversed when the inflammation resolves [16]. There is evidence that inflammation may affect coupling associated with bone resorption induced by periodontal pathogens [9]. Bone coupling in periodontal disease is not balanced. Although it is obvious that there is less bone formation following bone resorption the mechanisms responsible for this observation have only recently been investigated. It has been shown that activation of the adaptive active immune response by a periodontal pathogen inhibits bone formation following bone resorption [17]. One mechanism through which this occurs is due to the impact of the adaptive immune response on bone cells. It has been proposed that activation of the adaptive immune response causes cell death through a process that involves FOXO1 nuclear translocation [17]. Furthermore, by deleting the apoptotic gene caspase-3 in mice the amount of bone coupling following resorp-

tion induced by *Porphyromonas gingivalis* increases [18]. This demonstrates the concept that inflammation may interfere with coupling in periodontal disease through a process of inducing death of osteoblasts or their precursors.

Another mechanism through which inflammation could affect the coupling process in the periodontium is by reducing the expression of bone-promoting factors as has been shown in diabetes-linked experimental periodontitis [16]. Factors that were suppressed by inflammation include TGF-β_1, BMP-2, BMP-6 and FGF-2, all of which are involved in stimulating new bone or connective formation. This is linked to the level of inflammation since the amount of new bone formation increases when TNF is inhibited. Moreover, inhibition of TNF has demonstrable cellular events on bone including reduced apoptosis and increased proliferation of bone-lining cells that resulted in an increase in osteoblast numbers [16]. Thus, high levels of TNF affect a number of cellular parameters that can prevent normal coupling in addition to stimulating bone loss through osteoclastogenesis.

The resolution of inflammation is an active process regulated by different pro-resolving molecules such as lipoxins and resolvins [19]. They regulate the inflammation by limiting the migration of PMNS to the site of the inflammation and by promoting the macrophage uptake of apoptotic cells as in the case of lipoxins. The benefit is to promote regeneration of periodontal tissue. Furthermore, RvE1 treatment in rabbits has been associated with restoration of interproximal tissue and bone that were lost during periodontal disease [19].

Overall, the innate and immune response caused by the periodontal pathogens invasion leads to high levels of inflammation producing cytokines expression leading to bone resorption through osteoclasts. Cytokines produced by Th2 cells and Tregs such as IL-4 and IL-10 have the opposite effect stimulating of tissue inhibitors of matrix metalloproteinases and OPG as well as restrict inflammatory cytokine production (fig. 3).

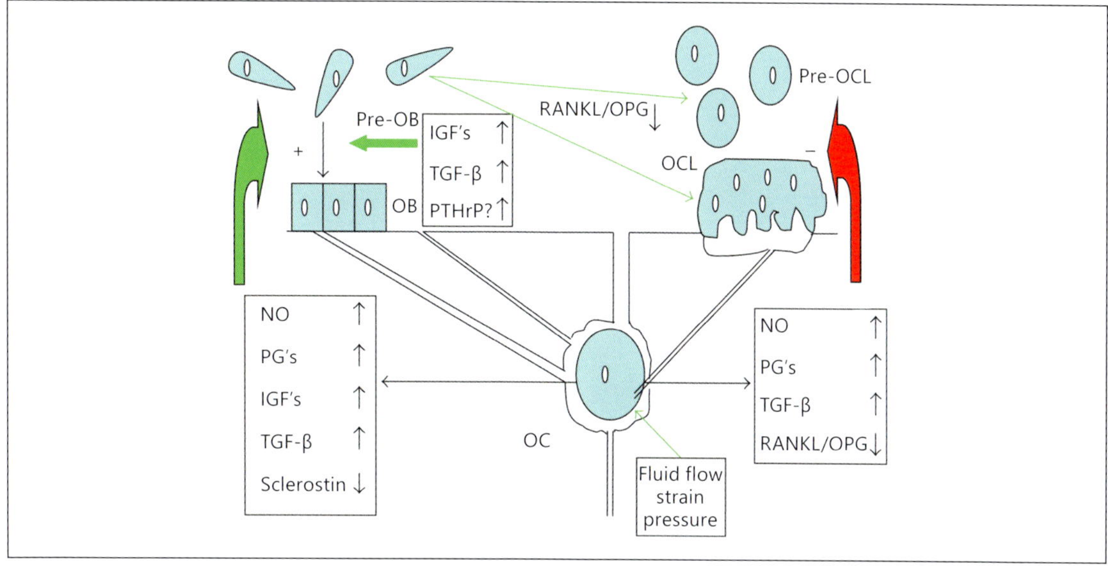

Fig. 4. Mechanotransduction in bone. OC = Osteocyte; OB = osteoblast; OCL = osteoclast; Pre-OB = preosteoblast; Pre-OCL = preosteoclast; PGs = prostaglandin (E_2 and I); RANKL = receptor-activating NFκB-ligand; OPG = osteoprotegerin; IGF = insulin-like growth factor; TGF = transforming growth factor; Scl = sclerostin; PTHrP = parathyroid hormone related peptide. Osteocytes sense the fluid flow induced by loading in the lacunocanalicular system; this signal modulates the secretion in the bone microenvironment of factors which can increase bone remodeling while stimulating osteoblast differentiation and activity (green arrows) and decreasing osteoclast activity (red arrow), resulting locally in a positive bone balance. From Bergmann et al. [22], reprinted with permission.

Bone Remodeling in Microgravity and Disuse

Mechanical forces are essential to maintain skeletal integrity. Long-term disuse, which includes the effects of paralysis due to spinal cord injury, long-term exposure to microgravity in space or tightly restricted mobility during bed rest have non-weight bearing periods that lead to compromised bone architecture, loss of mineral density and reduced bone mechanical properties [20, 21]. Disuse or microgravity leads to increased skeletal fragility, elevating fracture risk. Prolonged exposure to microgravity causes a 1–2% loss of bone mass per month, predominantly in the load-bearing regions of the legs and lumbar spine. It is also reported that space flight is associated with rapid decreases of bone formation makers with concomitant increases in markers of bone resorption. The loss of bone may be larger in regions that are rich in trabecular bone and less in regions rich in compact or cortical bone [21].

Unlike disuse, normally mechanical loading has a positive effect on bone formation and a negative effect on bone resorption. Osteocytes are sensitive to biomechanical stress, particularly to fluid flow and shear stress induced by loading in the lacunocanalicular system. Mechanical loading stimuli increase nitric oxide (NO), prostaglandins (PGs), IGF and TGF-β and induce a decrease in sclerostin expression by osteocytes (fig. 4). Each of these has a positive effect on osteoblast differentiation and activity. The increasing of NO, PGs and TGF-β and decreasing of RANKL/OPG by osteocytes also leads to a negative effect on osteoclast differentiation and activity. Mechanical deformations of osteoblasts can also lead to the generation of signals with increasing of IGF, TGF-β and parathyroid hormone-related peptide, which increase osteoblast proliferation at certain stages of differentiation. In addition, mechanical tensile stain decreases the expression of RANKL and OPG by osteoblast-like cells and osteocytes which causes a decrease in bone loss [22]. Thus, osteocytes sense mechanical stress and generate signals that enhance the generation of osteoblasts and bone formation (green arrows in fig. 4) and decrease osteoclast activity (red arrow in fig. 4), resulting in signals that enhance bone mass.

Microgravity or the effects of bone disuse has the opposite effect, increasing the RANKL/OPG ratio to enhance osteoclastogenesis [20, 21]. Bone marrow cultures of spinal cord-injured rats express higher levels of RANKL mRNA and slightly lower OPG levels than control rats [23]. Under weightlessness conditions there is upregulation of IL-6, which can lead to greater osteoclast formation. It has been reported that microgravity may cause sympathetic nervous system traffic that leads to greater osteoclast differentiation and activity. A similar result was found in disuse osteopenia. Elevated sympathetic stimulation or treatment with β-agonists stimulates osteoclast differentiation and activity, leading to increased bone resorption [21].

In disuse bone loss, osteoblastogenesis is inhibited by reduced differentiation from mesenchymal stem cells and by decreasing the function of the mature osteoblasts. Microgravity inhibits the proliferation of bone marrow stem cells and increases the rate of adipogenesis. The latter may be due to downregulation of Runx2 an important regulator of osteoblast differentiation and the upregulation of PPAR-γ, which controls adipogenesis [23, 24]. In disuse, bone loss formation of osteoblasts is inhibited through reduced expression of immediate early growth genes, such as cox-2, c-myc, bcl2, TGF-β_1, bFGF (FGF-2), BMP-4 and proliferating cell nuclear antigen. Decreasing the activity of the inducible cyclooxygenase, leads to prohibit prostaglandin synthesis [23, 24]. Phosphorylation events in the mitogen-activated protein kinase pathway and Runx2 activation are re-

duced in bone disuse and may contribute to reduced osteoblast proliferation and differentiation. Another avenue through which disuse may reduce osteoblast activity and differentiation is by suppressing the activity of RhoA (Ras homolog gene family, member A). When RhoA is inhibited there is a reduction in formation of actin cytoskeleton stress fibers and a delay in cell cycle progression [25, 26]. Local production of parathyroid hormone-related peptide is reduced by bone disuse. This has a negative effect on bone formation since it represents reduction of a positive signal for bone formation, parathyroid hormone-related peptide [22].

An alternative mechanism through which the absence of mechanical force may affect bone is through osteocyte expression of sclerostin. In bone disuse, sclerostin expression increases. Sclerostin binds to the Wnt receptor LRP5/6 and inhibits Wnt signaling. As a result, the β-catenin pathway is not activated, which is significant since β-catenin is an important modulator of pro-osteogenic transcription factors. In support of this sclerostin-deficient mice do not exhibit bone loss from hind limb unloading. This highlights that sclerostin is necessary for bone loss to occur in disuse. Thus by inhibiting Wnt, sclerostin reduces proliferation and differentiation, and stimulates apoptosis of osteoblasts and osteocytes [23, 24].

Bone disuse or microgravity increases production of RANKL and macrophage colony-stimulating factor by osteocytes. Osteocytes may also recruit osteoclast precursors and enhance bone resorption [23, 24]. Thus, in addition to having a negative effect on bone formation, disuse or microgravity has a positive effect on bone loss. Approximately 70% disuse bone loss is attributable to decreased bone formation and 30% to increased bone resorption [27]. Since disuse osteoporosis is due to non-weight-bearing, functional exercise is a primary nonpharmaceutical therapy. Local exercise provides bone with stimuli to generate signals that promote bone formation. Artificial gravity has a similar effect.

References

1 Lecart MP, Reginster JY: Current options for the management of postmenopausal osteoporosis. Expert Opin Pharmacother 2011;12:2533–2552.
2 Pacifici R: Estrogen deficiency, T cells and bone loss. Cell Immunol 2008;252:68–80.
3 Chang J, Wang Z, Tang E, et al: Inhibition of osteoblastic bone formation by nuclear factor-kappaB. Nat Med 2009; 15:682–689.
4 Lewiecki EM: New targets for intervention in the treatment of postmenopausal osteoporosis. Nat Rev Rheumatol 2011; 7:631–638.
5 Karmakar S, Kay J, Gravallese EM: Bone damage in rheumatoid arthritis: mechanistic insights and approaches to prevention. Rheum Dis Clin North Am 2010;36:385–404.
6 Maruotti N, Grano M, Colucci S, d'Onofrio F, Cantatore FP: Osteoclastogenesis and arthritis. Clin Exp Med 2011;11:137–145.
7 Walsh NC, Gravallese EM: Bone remodeling in rheumatic disease: a question of balance. Immunol Rev 2010;233:301–312.
8 Szekanecz Z, Koch AE, Tak PP: Chemokine and chemokine receptor blockade in arthritis, a prototype of immune-mediated inflammatory diseases. Neth J Med 2011;69:356–366.
9 Graves DT, Li J, Cochran DL: Inflammation and uncoupling as mechanisms of periodontal bone loss. J Dent Res 2010; 90:143–153.
10 Graves DT, Oates T, Garlet GP: Review of osteoimmunology and the host response in endodontic and periodontal lesions. J Oral Microbiol 2011;3:5304.
11 Scott DA, Krauss J: Neutrophils in periodontal inflammation. Front Oral Biol 2012;15:56–83.
12 Xiao W, Wang Y, Pacios S, Li S, Graves DT: Cellular and molecular aspects of bone remodeling. Monogr Oral Sci 2012, in press.
13 Garlet GP, Martins W Jr, Ferreira BR, Milanezi CM, Silva JS: Patterns of chemokines and chemokine receptors expression in different forms of human periodontal disease. J Periodontal Res 2003;38:210–217.
14 Jin Q, Cirelli JA, Park CH, et al: RANKL inhibition through osteoprotegerin blocks bone loss in experimental periodontitis. J Periodontol 2007;78:1300–1308.
15 Giannobile WV: Host-response therapeutics for periodontal diseases. J Periodontol 2008;79:1592–1600.
16 Pacios S, Kang J, Galicia J, et al: Diabetes aggravates periodontitis by limiting repair through enhanced inflammation. FASEB J 2012;26:1423–1430.
17 Behl Y, Siqueira M, Ortiz J, et al: Activation of the acquired immune response reduces coupled bone formation in response to a periodontal pathogen. J Immunol 2008;181:8711–8718.
18 Al-Mashat HA, Kandru S, Liu R, Behl Y, Desta T, Graves DT: Diabetes enhances mRNA levels of proapoptotic genes and caspase activity, which contribute to impaired healing. Diabetes 2006;55:487–495.
19 Hasturk H, Kantarci A, Van Dyke TE: Paradigm shift in the pharmacological management of periodontal diseases. Front Oral Biol 2012;15:160–176.
20 Tamma R, Colaianni G, Camerino C, et al: Microgravity during spaceflight directly affects in vitro osteoclastogenesis and bone resorption. FASEB J 2009;23:2549–2554.
21 Bloomfield SA: Disuse osteopenia. Curr Osteoporos Rep 2010;8:91–97.
22 Bergmann P, Body JJ, Boonen S, et al: Loading and skeletal development and maintenance. J Osteoporos 2010;2011:786752.
23 Huang Y, Dai ZQ, Ling SK, et al: Gravity, a regulation factor in the differentiation of rat bone marrow mesenchymal stem cells. J Biomed Sci 2009;16:87.
24 Hughes JM, Petit MA: Biological underpinnings of Frost's mechanostat thresholds: the important role of osteocytes. J Musculoskelet Neuronal Interact 2010; 10:128–135.
25 Meyers VE, Zayzafoon M, Douglas JT, McDonald JM: RhoA and cytoskeletal disruption mediate reduced osteoblastogenesis and enhanced adipogenesis of human mesenchymal stem cells in modeled microgravity. J Bone Miner Res 2005;20:1858–1866.
26 Nabavi N, Khandani A, Camirand A, et al: Effects of microgravity on osteoclast bone resorption and osteoblast cytoskeletal organization and adhesion. Bone 2011;49:965–974.
27 Sievänen H: Immobilization and bone structure in humans. Arch Biochem Biophys 2010;503:146–152.
28 Takayanagi H: Osteoimmunology and the effects of the immune system on bone. Nat Rev Rheumatol 2009;5:667–676.

Dana Graves
Department of Periodontics, University of Pennsylvania
240 S. 40th St., Levy 122
Philadelphia, PA 19104 (USA)
E-Mail dtgraves@dental.upenn.edu

Kantarci A, Will L, Yen S (eds): Tooth Movement. Front Oral Biol. Basel, Karger, 2016, vol 18, pp 28–35
DOI: 10.1159/000351897

Regional Acceleratory Phenomenon

Carlalberta Verna

Department of Orthodontics, School of Dentistry, University of Aarhus, Aarhus, Denmark

Abstract

The regional acceleratory phenomenon (RAP) is a tissue reaction to a noxious stimulus that increases the healing capacities of the affected tissues. It is typical not only of hard tissues such as bone and cartilage, but also of soft tissues. The RAP is characterized by acceleration of the normal cellular activities, as an 'SOS' phenomenon of the body that has to respond to the new perturbation. In the alveolar bone, the RAP is characterized, at a cellular level, by increased activation of the basic multicellular units (BMUs), thereby increasing the remodeling space. At the tissue level, the RAP is characterized by the production of woven bone, with the typical unorganized pattern, that will be reorganized into lamellar bone at a later stage. In the alveolar bone, the RAP occurs typically in the healing process of the alveolar sockets after tooth extraction, in periodontal disease, after surgery and trauma and during orthodontic tooth movement. In relation to orthodontic tooth movement, the RAP can be seen as a tissue response to the mechanical cyclical perturbation that induces the formation of microdamage that has to be removed to avoid their accumulation and the following bone failure. The adaptation to the new orthodontically induced mechanical environment is ensured by an increased activation of the BMU that returns to normal levels after few months.

The regional acceleratory phenomenon (RAP) is a tissue reaction to different noxious stimuli that was first described as a general entity by Harold Frost [1]. The RAP is characterized by an acceleration of normal ongoing tissue processes and involves both soft and hard tissue. It is a ubiquitous and general postinjury phenomenon that does not solely occur in the skeleton, but also in the abdominal viscera, in the intracranial and thoracic cavities, and in the soft tissue of the nasopharyngeal and oral cavities [2].

A RAP can be evoked in the normal body by any regional noxious stimulus and is directly proportional to the magnitude and nature of the stimulus. The noxious stimuli include infections of soft tissues, bone and joints, crushing injuries, contusions, fractures of any kind, surgical interventions, acute peripheral denervation and acute paralysis of central origin, and most noninfectious inflammatory processes.

Once evoked, the vital processes accelerate above normal values. The metabolism and the activities of the differentiated cells, the activities of the precursor cells, the differentiation of cells, longitudinal and transversal growth of bone and cartilage, together with bone multicellular unit (BMU)-based remodeling of lamellar bone are all activities that are affected by the RAP on bone tissues, such as woven bone, lamellar bone, spongiosa and compacta [2].

Bone remodeling occurs in discrete locations and consists of a sequence of resorption and subsequent formation activities that are spatially and temporally coupled, in a cyclical sequence. Remodeling allows bone to adjust to mechanical stresses by repairing fatigue damages and is influenced by the action of hormones and cytokines [3–5]. The types of cells managing the bone remodeling cycle form the BMU [2].

The different cells of this team act in a specific sequence composed by 4 phases: activation, resorption, reversal and formation. In the activation phase, bone-lining cells become cuboidal in shape, preosteoblasts, and present receptor activator of nuclear factor K (RANK) ligand (RANKL), on the cell surface. RANKL interacts with RANK present on the cell membrane of preosteoclasts from the bone marrow and activates their fusion and differentiation into mature multinucleated osteoclasts which resorb bone. Bone resorption lasts for about 2 weeks, after which the osteoclasts undergo programmed cell death or apoptosis. At the reversal phase, mononucleated phagocyte cells complete the resorption and deepen the lacunae [6]. Subsequent bone formation requires the differentiation of preosteoblasts into osteoblasts. In the reversal phase, preosteoblasts migrate into the resorbed cavity and differentiate later into osteoblasts. Mature osteoblasts secrete osteoprotegerin, a free-floating decoy receptor belonging to the tumor necrosis factor family. It can bind the RANKL, thus preventing the further activation of the preosteoclasts. The border between the resorbed old bone and the newly formed bone is called the cement line or reversal line. The secreting osteoblasts secrete layers of osteoid, and the resorption cavity is slowly refilled and mineralized in about 3–4 months. The new bone consists in closely packed mineral crystals whose density subsequently increases throughout time.

The remodeling space, i.e. the sum of all of the active bone-remodeling units in the skeleton at a given time, increases during a RAP. The acceleration of local bone turnover is characterized by an increased intake of bone-seeking isotopes and radiographically by areas of less bone density. The duration of the RAP depends on the tissue and on the entity of the noxious stimulus; in bone a RAP following, for example, a femoral fracture lasts between 4 and 8 months, but it may last longer for severer stimuli and is longer for adults than in growing patients.

The RAP may represent an 'SOS' mechanism that potentiates the healing and local tissue defense activities against infection and mechanical abuse, as a sign of survival of the species to the competitive environment. In this perspective, the RAP is a necessary step for proper bone healing and, as a consequence, if a RAP fails to develop, healing may be delayed and infections may occur more easily [7].

In the mandible and in the maxilla, the RAP occurs after tooth extraction, following fractures and surgical procedures and implant placement, in periodontal disease and during orthodontic tooth movement. In all the above-mentioned circumstances, in fact, the alveolar or basal bones are submitted to a noxious stimulus, whether mechanical or infectious.

Concerning mechanical stimuli, the RAP occurs mainly under specific loading circumstances. Frost [8] described the occurrence of remodeling, modeling and RAP according to the loading history of bone through the mechanostat theory, thus elucidating the complex concepts of bone biomechanics. Bone modeling activities are driven by dynamic loads above and below the normal physiological range. The ultimate strength of bone is ~25,000 microstrain units ($\mu\varepsilon$), and the normal physiological range of bone loading is ~200–2,500 $\mu\varepsilon$. With this background, four 'mechanical usage windows' are identified, and, according to the mechanical loading, different modeling, remodeling or RAP activities prevail.

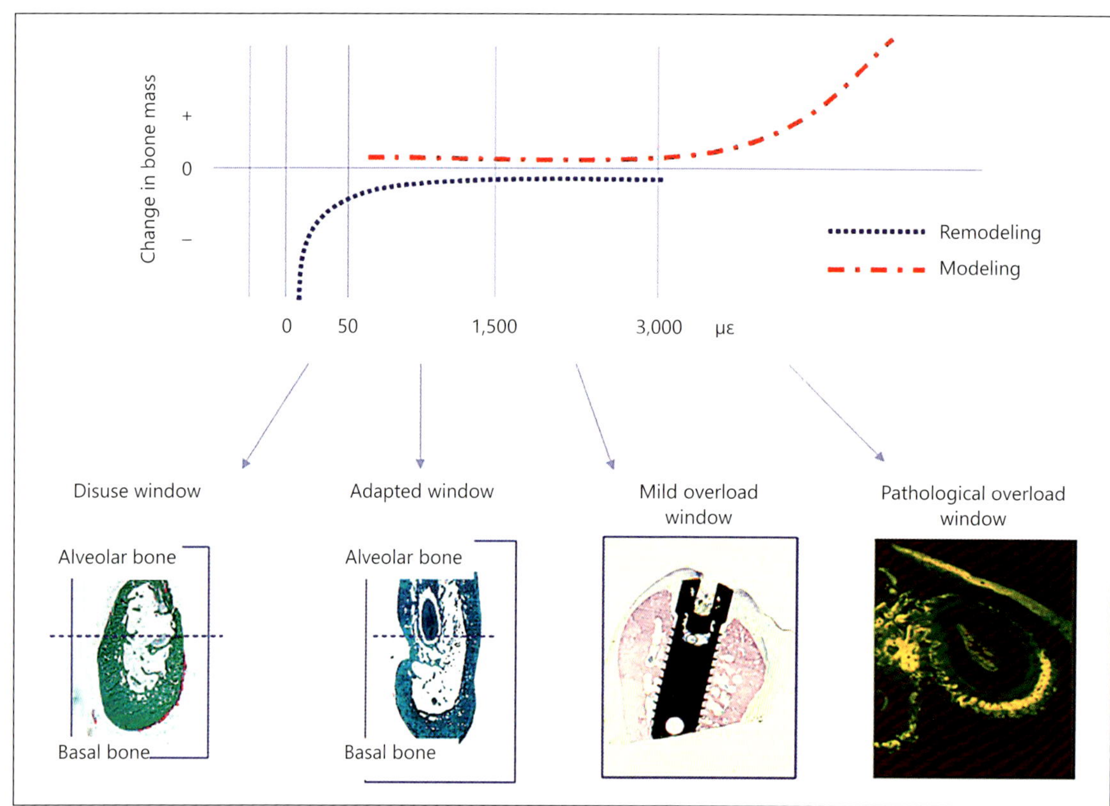

Fig. 1. The mechanostat for dentists. The upper part shows the graph of bone activities in relation to the mechanical history. The four mechanical usage windows are described in the text. Bone turnover is increased with negative bone balance (–) in the disuse windows, as in edentulous areas. Bone balance is maintained in the adapted and in the mild overload windows, with a tendency towards new bone formation via surface hypertrophy, as shown in cases of dental implants. New bone formation and increased activation of BMUs is seen in the pathological overload windows, as following the application of an orthodontic load with woven bone formation. In the lower part of the figure, histological sections showing an atrophic mandibular human specimen, a histological section of a human mandible with load-bearing teeth, a section of a dental implant and the surrounding alveolar bone, and a section of maxillary alveolar bone of rat showing (yellow marks) increased formation of woven bone following the application of an orthodontic load (with permission from Libra Ortodonzia and reprinted from Verna et al. [29], with permission from Elsevier).

In the so-called 'disuse windows' strains are below 50 με, well below the physiological range. BMU formation in this window increases with negative bone balance occurrence and consequent weakening of bone. No microdamage or RAP occurs at this strain level. The case of disuse atrophy following immobilization is the typical clinical situation reflecting unloading of bone. The related clinical situation for dentists is seen in the alveolar ridge atrophy observed in edentulous areas (fig. 1). In the so-called 'adapted window' the typical bone strain ranges between 50 and 1,500 με, with normal formation of BMU and balance between resorption and formation. This is the case of the alveolar bone with healthy periodontium loaded by teeth (fig. 1).

In the so-called 'mild overload windows' the peak bone strain ranges from 1,500 to about 3,000 με. The creation of BMU stays near the normal, no RAP occurs, while little new microdamage arises. The generation of a macro- and a consequent microcrack is considered a triggering factor for the initiation of a remodeling cycle, whose role it is to avoid the accumulation of cracks and the consequent mechanical failure [4, 9, 10]. However, the remodeling ensures an efficient removal of fatigue damage, and bone structural integrity is maintained. When the peak strain exceeds 2,500 $\mu\varepsilon$, subperiosteal hypertrophy builds bone mass to reduce the surface strain. In the case of alveolar bone, an example is the dental implant, where bone adapts to the new mechanical pattern. Formation drift at this bone strain level usually results in lamellar bone (fig. 1).

In the 'pathological overload window', bone is repetitively loaded at strains which are above 3,000 $\mu\varepsilon$. BMU formation increases and the RAP occurs, consequently increasing bone turnover rate. The newly formed bone is woven bone, and the risk of anarchic bone resorption occurs. Fatigue damage accumulates more rapidly than it can be repaired, and the bone is at risk for stress fracture. It is the case of bone weakened by a cyst or tumors. The mass and orientation of bone seems therefore to be molded through disuse atrophy and overload hypertrophy [11]. It is interesting to consider the mechanical loading of the alveolar bone that occurs via the application of an orthodontic force bone in the light of the bone strain history and Frost's mechanostat theory.

The mechanical loading has traditionally been described as compression and tension, the attention being commonly focused on the stress and strain distribution within the viscoelastic structure of the periodontal ligament. However, the deformation of the periodontal ligament (PDL) does not mirror the deformation that occurs in the surrounding bone. A finite element study has shown that the transfer mechanism of orthodontic loads through the alveolar supporting structures cannot be explained in terms of compression and tension. Considering the properties of the PDL as nonlinear, tension was more predominant than compression, and the alveolar bone

situated in the 'traditional' compressive area is loaded significantly less than the bone on the tension side. Both compressive and tensile strains are present in the area from which the tooth is moving and no tension and very little compressive strains are present in the bone in the direction of the force [12]. In the areas from which the tooth is moving, the tensile stresses produced by the pulling of the PDL fibers are transformed into compressive hoop stresses similarly to the principle of the roman arch. Therefore, both tensile and compressive stresses coexist on the 'tension' side. On the 'pressure' side the fibers of the PDL become curled up, and practically no stresses are transferred onto the alveolar wall (fig. 2). Consequently, the hoop stresses are low as well, and the overall stress concentration becomes much lower as on the 'tension' side. It seems therefore that the generally accepted concept, which suggests that compression leads to bone resorption and that tension leads to bone formation, is questionable, and a more reasonable biological model seems to be the one involving loading/nonloading of the alveolar support structures. In a loading history perspective [13], this situation can be associated with the disuse window, when bone senses a decreased mechanical loading. Bone turnover increases, and resorption activities will prevail (fig. 2). However, this represents the very first initiation of the bony reaction.

Further application of an orthodontic load generates bone reactions that lead to an adaptation to the new mechanical environment, achieving progressive balance between resorption and formation, as in the 'adapted and mild overload windows' (fig. 2). This ensures tooth movement with bone, i.e. the movement of the tooth surrounded by the alveolar bone.

When sustained mechanical load is applied by some orthodontic appliance, the 'pathological overload window' may be reached. Hyalinization of the PDL, ischemia-induced necrosis of the lining cells and microdamage of the bone in the direction of the force will lead to increased BMU

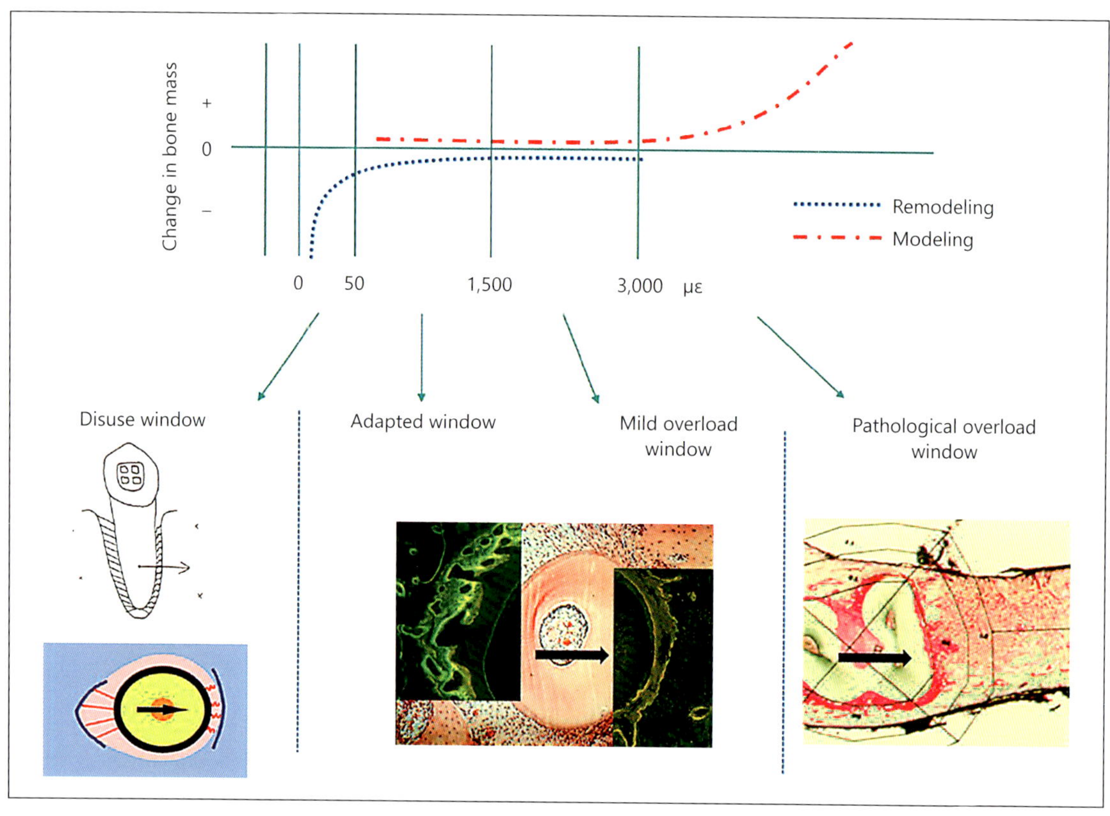

Fig. 2. The loading history of the alveolar bone following the application of an orthodontic load. For the description of the strain windows, see figure 1. At the very initial stage, the tension of the periodontal fibers in the direction of the force decreases, as schematized in the lower left pictures. The sudden change in loading activates the BMUs, as in a disuse window. Tooth movement occurs with the surrounding alveolar bone in the adapted and in the mild overload window. Bone-resorptive and -formative activities are in balance. The lower middle picture is a histological section of a tooth whose PDL space is thinner in the direction of the force and wider on the opposite side. In green, the related bone formation activities are presented: small amounts of bone formation in the direction of the force and large amounts on the opposite side. In the pathological overload window, a clear RAP is observed in the direction of the force. Here a horizontal section of a mandibular tooth of a monkey shows woven bone ahead of the tooth in the direction of the force (with permission of Libra Ortodonzia, and the E.H. Angle Education and Research Foundation).

activation frequency and increased remodeling space [7, 14] (fig. 3). In 2004, Verna et al. [15] showed a significant increase in crack density in the direction of force application after 1 day of treatment, and it is therefore tempting to hypothesize that the response is mediated by a transient increase in microdamage of the bone supporting orthodontically loaded teeth [16]. The presence of accelerated bone remodeling following the application of an orthodontic load is well described [17–19]. Synchronized initiation of numerous BMUs characterizes bone turnover at both sides of pressure and tension, and the remodeling of the whole alveolar bone is induced by mechanical force in addition to conventional changes of the bone adjacent to the PDL [20]. In the direction of the force, bone formation has also been demonstrated [21, 22], and bone resorption on the so-called tension side was found [22, 23]. A RANKL-RANK mechanism has been shown to be present

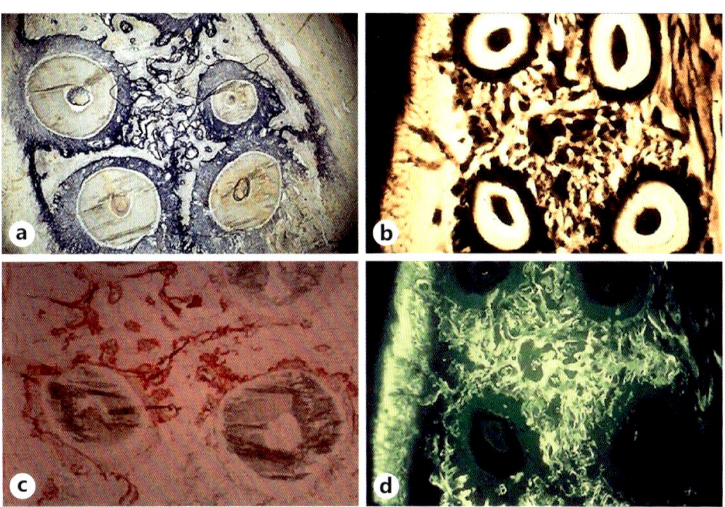

Fig. 3. Alkaline (**a**) and acid (**c**) phosphatase staining of an interradicular area of a rat molar after the application of an orthodontic load of 25 g for 2 weeks. The 10-μm-thick sections are taken consecutively. Please observe the positive staining for both anabolic (**a**) and catabolic (**c**) activities, supporting the presence of a RAP after the application of an orthodontic load. The microradiographic image of the same samples (**b**) reveals decreased bone density and the formation of woven bone. The intensity of vowen bone formation activities is detected by the uptake of tetracycline labeling, as depicted in **d** (with permission from Libra Ortodonzia and the Italian Society of Orthodontics).

in the PDL and to be straightened by mechanical load [24]. Local delivery of RANKL or of osteoprotegerin has been shown to accelerate or reduce tooth movement, respectively [25–27].

The increased number of BMUs activated per time unit is reflected in a larger amount of bone surface covered by active bone-resorptive and bone-formative cells (fig. 3). Increased apposition of woven bone is observed in the interradicular area of rat molars loaded by 25 cN but is also observed in front of the alveolar socket in the direction towards which tooth movement occurs, together with the periosteal apposition surface (fig. 3, 4) [14, 23, 28, 29]. As long as alveolar bone cells persist, the stress leads to a strain-generated RAP phenomenon, otherwise failure is expected. The initial woven bone is reorganized in time into lamellar bone. The intensity of the response gradually decreases as the distance from the involved site increases. Verna et al. [29] found, in an animal study, that the RAP occurs not only around the teeth directly loaded with the orthodontic appliance, but also at distant sites.

It is important therefore to stress that the level of loading plays an important role in the final treatment results. This is particularly true where

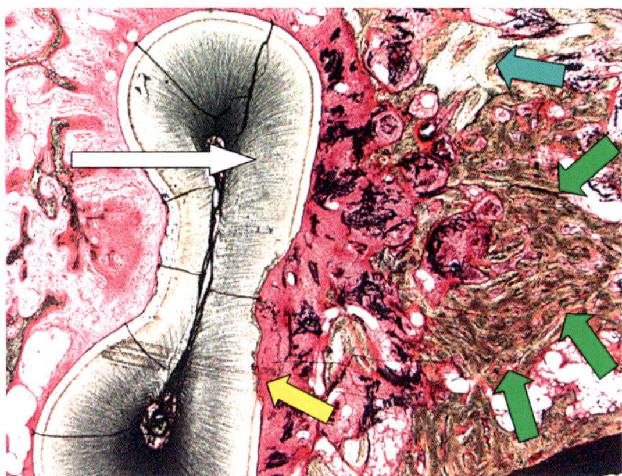

Fig. 4. Transverse section of monkey mandible after the application of an orthodontic load in the direction of the white arrow. Note the formation of woven bone in the direction of the force (green arrows) as a sign of tissue repair (RAP). Old bone close to the cortex is also present (blue arrow), together with root resorption in the direction of the force (yellow arrow) (reprinted from Verna et al. [33], with permission of Wiley-Blackwell).

tooth movement has to be performed in areas where the ratio between cortical and trabecular bone is particularly high, as in the symphyseal area. Since the turnover of cortical bone is lower than the one of trabecular bone, the 'SOS' mechanism of the RAP may occur less effectively with a higher risk for lack of balance between resorption and formation.

Some nonmechanical factors (genes, hormones, vitamins, minerals, drugs and other agents) seem to be able to modify the minimum effective strain thresholds listed above, thus explaining the onset of some diseases [30]. This may also be the explanation of the accelerated tooth movement observed under high turnover conditions [31].

Orthodontic tooth movement can therefore be seen as a modified skeletal wound healing and adaptation, typified by an increased bone remodeling response in addition to an elevated formation of woven bone. In this perspective, the biological principle of the RAP is exploited in surgically facilitated orthodontics [32].

References

1 Frost HM: The regional acceleratory phenomenon: a review. Henry Ford Hosp Med J 1983;31:3–9.
2 Frost HM: Intermediary Organization of the Skeleton. Boca Raton, CRC Press, 1986, vol I, II.
3 Frost HM: A brief review for orthopedic surgeons: fatigue damage (microdamage) in bone (its determinants and clinical implications). J Orthop Sci 1998;3:272–281.
4 Burr DB: Remodeling and the repair of fatigue damage. Calcif Tissue Int 1993;53(suppl 1):S75–S80.
5 Mori S, Burr DB: Increased intracortical remodeling following fatigue damage. Bone 1993;14:103–109.
6 Eriksen EF, Gundersen HJ, Melsen F, Mosekilde L: Reconstruction of the formative site in iliac trabecular bone in 20 normal individuals employing a kinetic model for matrix and mineral apposition. Metab Bone Dis Relat Res 1984;5:243–252.
7 Frost HM: Wolff's law and bone's structural adaptations to mechanical usage: an overview for clinicians. Angle Orthod 1994;64.175–188.
8 Frost HM: Bone 'mass' and the 'mechanostat': a proposal. Anat Rec 1987;219:1–9.
9 Verborgt O, Gibson GJ, Schaffler MB: Loss of osteocyte integrity in association with microdamage and bone remodeling after fatigue in vivo. J Bone Miner Res 2000;15:60–67.
10 Noble B: Bone microdamage and cell apoptosis. Eur Cell Mater 2003;6:46–55.
11 Roberts WE, Huja S, Roberts JA: Bone modeling: biomechanics, molecular mechanisms, and clinical perspectives. Semin Orthodont 2004;10:123–161.
12 Cattaneo PM, Dalstra M, Melsen B: The finite element method: a tool to study orthodontic tooth movement. J Dent Res 2005;84:428–433.
13 Frost HM: Bone's mechanostat: a 2003 update. Anat Rec A Discov Mol Cell Evol Biol 2003;275:1081–1101.
14 Melsen B: Biological reaction of alveolar bone to orthodontic tooth movement. Angle Orthod 1999;69:131–138.
15 Verna C, Dalstra M, Lee TC, Cattaneo PM, Melsen B: Microcracks in the alveolar bone following orthodontic tooth movement: a morphological and morphometric study. Eur J Orthod 2004;26:459–467.
16 Roberts WE, Epker BN, Burr DB, Hartsfield JK Jr, Roberts JA: Remodeling of mineralized tissues. II. Control and pathophysiology. Semin Orthodont 2006;12:238–253.
17 Chambers TJ: The pathobiology of the osteoclast. J Clin Pathol 1985;38:241–252.
18 Rodan GA, Martin TJ: Role of osteoblasts in hormonal control of bone resorption – a hypothesis. Calcif Tissue Int 1981;33:349–351.
19 Baron R: Importance of the intermediate phases between resorption and formation in the measurement and understanding of the bone remodeling sequence; in Meunier PJ (ed): Bone Histomorphometry. Second International Workshop. Lyon, Armour Montagu, 1976, pp 179–183.
20 Tanne K, Nagataki T, Matsubara S, Kato J, Terada Y, Sibaguchi T, et al: Association between mechanical stress and bone remodeling. J Osaka Univ Dent Sch 1990;30:64–71.
21 King GJ, Keeling SD, Wronski TJ: Histomorphological and chemical study of alveolar bone turnover in response to orthodontic tipping; in Carlson DS, Goldstein SA (eds): Bone biodynamics in orthodontic and orthopedic treatment. Ann Arbor, Center for Human Growth and Development, 1992, pp 281–297.
22 Mohri T, Hanada K, Osawa H: Coupling of resorption and formation on bone remodeling sequence in orthodontic tooth movement: a histochemical study. J Bone Miner Metab 1991;9:57–69.
23 Zaffe D, Verna C: Acid and alkaline phosphatase activities in rat's alveolar bone experimentally loaded by orthodontical forces (abstract). Ital J Miner Electrol Metab 1995;9(suppl 1):11.
24 Ogasawara T, Yoshimine Y, Kiyoshima T, Kobayashi I, Matsuo K, Akamine A, et al: In situ expression of RANKL, RANK, osteoprotegerin and cytokines in osteoclasts of rat periodontal tissue. J Periodontal Res 2004;39:42–49.
25 Kanzaki H, Chiba M, Arai K, Takahashi I, Haruyama N, Nishimura M, et al: Local RANKL gene transfer to the periodontal tissue accelerates orthodontic tooth movement. Gene Ther 2006;13:678–685.
26 Kanzaki H, Chiba M, Takahashi I, Haruyama N, Nishimura M, Mitani H: Local OPG gene transfer to periodontal tissue inhibits orthodontic tooth movement. J Dent Res 2004;83:920–925.

27 Oshiro T, Shiotani A, Shibasaki Y, Sasaki T: Osteoclast induction in periodontal tissue during experimental movement of incisors in osteoprotegerin-deficient mice. Anat Rec 2002;266: 218–225.

28 Reitan K: Clinical and histologic observations on tooth movement during and after orthodontic treatment. Am J Orthod 1967;53:721–745.

29 Verna C, Zaffe D, Siciliani G: Histomorphometric study of bone reactions during orthodontic tooth movements in rats. Bone 1999;24:371–379.

30 Frost HM: From Wolff's law to the mechanostat: a new 'face' of physiology. J Orthop Sci 1998;3:282–286.

31 Verna C, Melsen B: Tissue reaction to orthodontic tooth movement in different metabolic conditions. Orthodont Craniofac Res 2003;6:155–163.

32 Baloul SS, Gerstenfeld LC, Morgan EF, Carvalho RS, Van Dyke TE, Kantarci A: Mechanism of action and morphologic changes in the alveolar bone in response to selective alveolar decortication-facilitated tooth movement. Am J Orthod Dentofacial Orthop 2011; 139:S83–S101.

33 Verna C, et al: Tissue reaction; in Melsen B (ed): Adult Orthodontics. Hoboken, Wiley-Blackwell, 2012.

Carlalberta Verna, DDS, PhD
Department of Orthodontics, School of Dentistry, University of Aarhus
Vennelyst boulevard 9
DK–8000 Aarhus-C (Denmark)
E-Mail carlalberta.verna@odontologi.au.dk

Kantarci A, Will L, Yen S (eds): Tooth Movement. Front Oral Biol. Basel, Karger, 2016, vol 18, pp 36–45
DOI: 10.1159/000351898

Tissue Reaction and Biomechanics

Birte Melsen

Section of Orthodontics, Department of Dentistry, Aarhus University, Aarhus, Denmark

Abstract

Tissue reaction to orthodontic force has been a subject of research with the purpose of providing the orthodontists with information necessary for the application of a force system that can generate a maximum of tooth movement and modeling of the alveolar process with a minimum of damage. Traditionally, the studies of bone biological reactions have been distinguishable from those performed by bone biologists. This has led to a controversy regarding both the terminology and perception of the reaction to mechanical perturbation. The present chapter, with its basis in bone biology, surveys the attempts by orthodontists to optimize the tissue reaction and shorten treatment time. © 2016 S. Karger AG, Basel

The interest in tissue reaction related to tooth movement dates back to the beginning of the 20th century and in spite of the presentation of many alternative models, the classic pressure-tension theory has prevailed and is still the theory found in most textbooks [1]. This does to some degree reflect a lack of communication between orthodontists and bone biologists, as the biologists have clearly demonstrated that osteocytes, which are considered the receptors of mechanical stimuli, are not able to differentiate between compression and tension, but are only sensitive to variation in strain leading to deformation of the cell membrane and the cytoskeleton [2, 3].

The interest in tissue reaction is first and foremost grounded in the fact that it is presumed that a better understanding will set the stage for the possibility of controlling the reaction to avoid damage to roots and periodontium and to shorten the treatment time.

Shortening of the treatment time has been attempted from time to time in the eighties by Yamasaki et al. [4] who injected prostaglandin and obtained an increased rate of tooth movement [5, 6] due to increased resorption activity. With the same purpose, Davidovitch et al. [7, 8] performed several animal experiments applying electric current to the appliance in cats and found increased staining for cyclic nucleotides, faster resorption at the anode on the compression site and enhancement of bone formation on the tension side near the cathode. There was, however, an apparent conflict between these results and electric potential measured when bending a long bone. Otter et al. [9] found that in the compressed area there was a negative potential leading to apposition. This conflict was later discussed by Melsen [10], who demonstrated increased bone density in the direction of the tooth movement. She suggested a new paradigm whereby the direct resorption was compared to the increase in the turnover (remodeling) leading to a negative balance occurring as a result of inactivity; in other words, too low strain values, whereas the indirect undermining resorption following the hyalinization could be perceived as a repair with the purpose to remove the necrotic tissues resulting from the local ischemia. With this explanation the tissue reaction generated by the application of orthodontic forces to a tooth would be in concordance with that of the bone's mechanostate described by Frost [3] (fig. 1). The new paradigm was further corroborated in a finite element model where Cattaneo and coworkers [11, 12] modeled the periodontal ligament with nonlinear properties thereby approximating the reality more than in previously described models which all considered the PDL as a solid (fig. 2). However, von Bohl and Kuijpers-Jagtman's group [5, 6] demonstrated that even with low forces, hyalinization can never be avoided. This statement was supported by the findings of Dalstra et al. [13], who studied the alveolar wall in 3D in synchrotron generated images. They found that the alveolar wall is a highly irregular structure with multiple extensions reaching into the PDL (fig. 3). As a consequence, even very low forces will generate strain values sufficient for the release of the cascade leading to the breaking down the alveolar wall [14].

When Long et al. [15] surveyed methods for enhancing rapid tooth movement they concluded that only corticotomy and dentoalveolar distractions are convincing methods. This could be explained by the increased turnover, a RAP phenomenon, occurring during the healing of a local trauma (discussed by Verna in this book). The principle that was introduced by the Wilcko brothers as 'Wilckodontics' involved full flap surgery, full thickness flap reflection, selective corticotomy and bone grafting [16, 17] around the teeth to be moved. A less invasive, but still effective modification of the corticision has later been

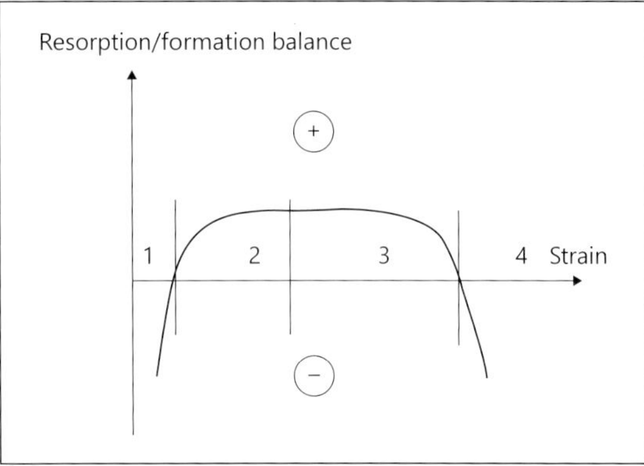

Fig. 1. Dependency of the balance between bone turnover and strain. With a low strain (1) inactivity, the balance is negative due to increased remodeling. When the strain is increasing, positive is obtained with the formation of lamellar bone (2), and with increasing strain the newly formed bone will be woven bone which will later remodel into lamellar bone. With even greater strain, the number of microfractures occurring will exceed the possibility of repair and this may lead to a negative balance. In relation to orthodontics, the high strain will result in ischemia and local necrosis. The indirect resorption can be perceived as a repair of this process.

suggested by Korean orthodontists [18], but only few randomized controlled studies controlling the effect have been published. The same principle was used for increasing the rate of canine retraction [19].

Whereas the tissue reaction to the enhancement of tooth movement by means of the RAP phenomena is well recognized, the mechanism behind the application of rare earth magnets seems to be different. In a rat experiment, Tomizuka demonstrated that the lag phase normally seen in relation to tooth movement did not occur, and a gradual recruitment of osteoclasts without hyalinization was seen. This may be the result of the force system, which in contrast to the conventional appliances starts at a low level and increases when the magnets are approximating. This principle has been used in relation to closure of open bites [20] but also recently in relation to functional appliances [21].

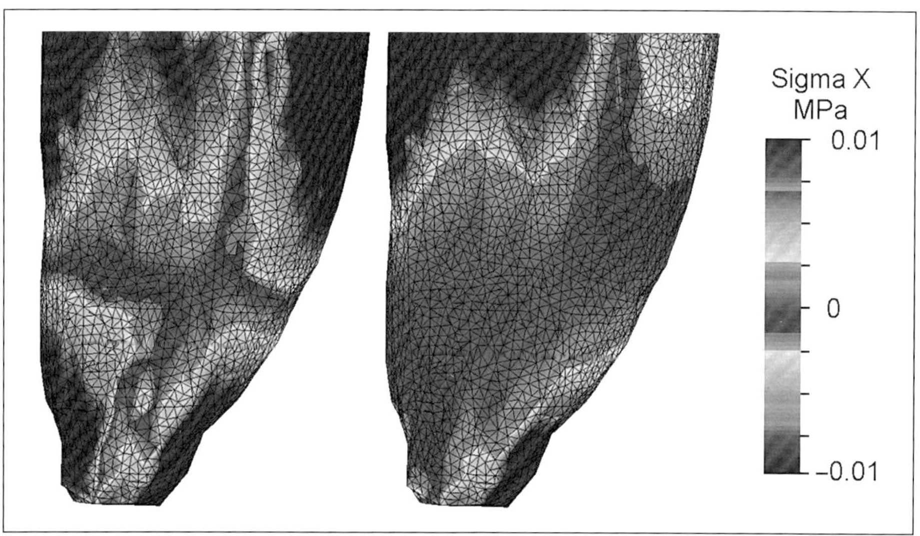

Fig. 2. Finite element models illustrating the strain on the alveolar wall the a premolar is loaded with a force generating controlled tipping. In the figure to the left the periodontal ligament is modeled as a solid which results in a compression of the marginal bone. In the image to the left, the periodontal ligament is modeled in a nonstrain is increasing on the so-called 'tension' site and that there is no compression of the bone in the direction of the force. From Cattaneo et al. [12].

Whereas the above-mentioned efforts to influence tissue reaction have been directed toward the enhancement of the tooth movement, a different approach to the reduction of the treatment time has focused on the hardware, brackets and wires. By changing the bracket design the manufactures have concentrated on the reduction of friction related to the sliding of the brackets on the wire. Despite the repeated demonstration of the fact that friction is only a minor part of resistance to sliding, the marketing of special brackets characterized by low friction has had a significant impact on orthodontics [22–24] and a large number of unsupported claims followed the introduction of the new brackets [25]. Evidence of an increased rate of treatment as a result of the use of specific brackets is, however, still missing and claims related to these brackets have been gradually refuted [26].

Yet another attempt to reduce treatment time has focused on force delivery. The question regarding continuous versus intermittent forces has already been addressed by Andersen et al. [27], who demonstrated that forces delivered from continuous wires would be perceived by the periodontium as intermittent due to the interaction with occlusal forces (fig. 4). Only rectangular stainless steel wires were able to mask the forces delivered from the occlusion. Lately, interest in force delivery and its possible influence on treatment time has led to the development of an appliance delivering vibration movements [28]. Preliminary experiments confirm that cyclic force delivery has a positive influence on treatment time [29]. The biological reaction was explained by an increased RANKL expression at the levels of fibroblasts and osteoclasts.

Independent of the approach and the model used for assessing the rate of tooth movement, whether human clinical studies or animal experiments, the result of all the different attempts to increase the rate of tooth movements have been characterized by a large inter-individual variation most likely to some degree explainable by

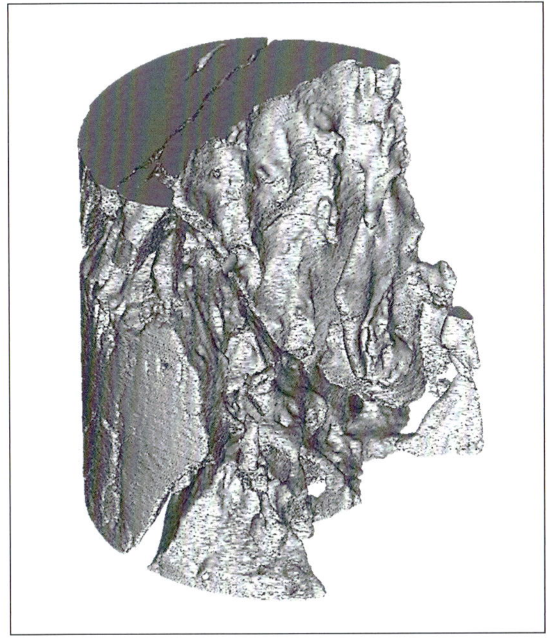

Fig. 3. Synchrotron image of a human alveolar wall illustrating the impressive irregularity of the alveolar wall allowing for the generation of sufficient strain for the formation of a hyalinization even with very low forces. From Dalstra et al. [14].

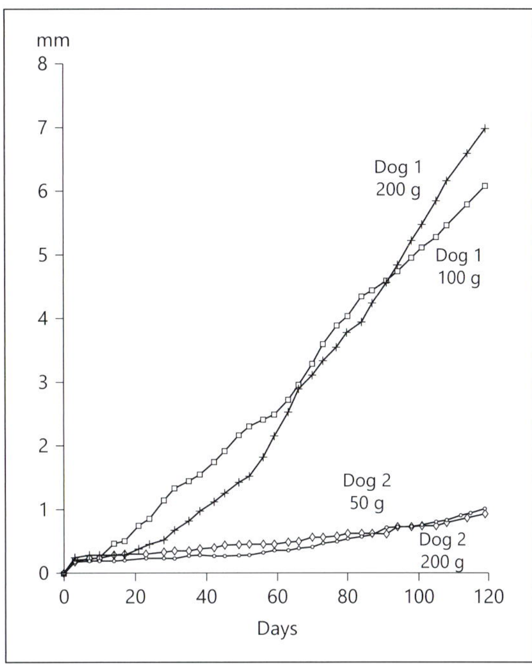

Fig. 5. Graphic image of tooth displacement in different dogs with different forces. The graph illustrates the interindividual difference and the lack of influence of variation in force level. From Pilon et al. [31].

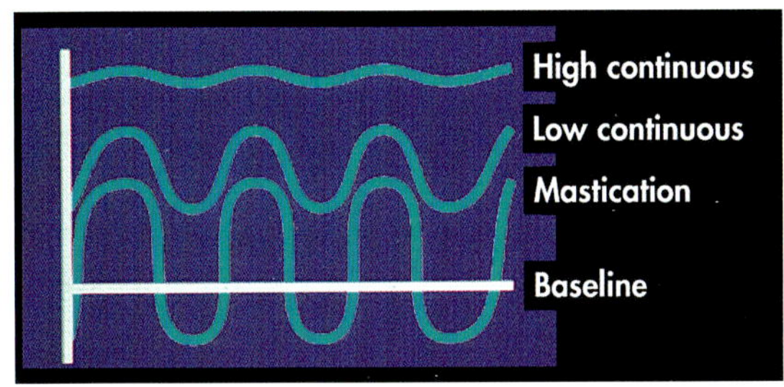

Fig. 4. Illustration of how continuous forces are influenced by occlusal forces.

inter-individual variation in bone turnover, which again [30] could reflect genetic differences. The inter-individual variation was demonstrated clearly in a dog experiment by Pilon et al. [31] and measurements carried out by Roberts et al. [32] when protracting a lower molar into edentulous space (fig. 5).

The orthodontic treatment time varies even more in relation to treatment of young growing children, who are often treated in a two-phase treatment, which prolongs the total treatment time, but not necessarily chair time. The discussion regarding one- or two-stage treatment is still ongoing, and while the treatment time will be dependent on growth and eruption of teeth in two-phase treatments this is not the case in the one-phase treatment. The early treatment does on the other hand seem to have a more profound skeletal influence [33].

In the growing patient growth and development is responsible for the major proportion of the treatment effect, and attempts to reduce treatment time should therefore only be performed in patients where growth does not interfere. When assessing the efficacy of the various approaches to reduce treatment time it is important that the groups are as homogenous as possible, and large enough to mask the confounder effect from the interindividual variation.

The reduction in treatment time was the focus of a recent survey by the group behind SureSmile®, Sachdeva et al. [34] compared the treatment time of 9,390 SureSmile patients with that of 2,945 conventionally treated patients and found that the SureSmile pool was treated for 15 months on an average compared to 23 months for the conventional group. The reduction in treatment time is higher than reported in any of the above-mentioned attempts to enhance the tooth movement. This may, however, to some degree, be a result of the design of the study. The SureSmile patients were most likely all one-phase treatment patients with full dentition and in spite of the large interindividual variation also in these groups (4–45 months) the differences between mean values turned out to be significant due to the large number of patients in each group. In addition, the conventional patients referred to in this study required a longer treatment time, 23 months, compared to those reported by other authors, e.g. Hamilton et al. [35]. Previously reported attempts to increase the rate of tooth movements have focused on the change in the local biological environment or on reducing the friction with the appliance. SureSmile treatment, on the other hand, focuses on the control of the movements of the individual teeth, which with the custommade computer-bend arches most likely will reduce the 'jiggling', or changing the direction of tooth movement which normally characterizes the standard straight wire treatment. This will certainly reduce the treatment time.

Standard treatments traditionally start with a leveling, which, in most cases, will lead to some undesirable tooth movements. In the case of variation in vertical position, a leveling arch will generate an extrusion and a buccal root torque on some teeth whereas the intrusion generated on the adjacent tooth will result in a lingual root torque. Correction of this difference in torque will, on the other hand, deliver adverse vertical forces all of which result in a considerable amount of 'jiggling', indicating that many teeth, if not all, will have to be displaced in different, often opposite, directions. An example of the leveling of incisors with vertical discrepancies is seen in figure 6. Another typical example would be the proclination of the central incisors in a patient with a class II division 2 malocclusion, which is often performed before retraction of the anterior teeth in an extraction case. It is, however, not only in extraction cases, that 'jiggling' occurs.

The shortest distance between two points, the position of a tooth before and at the treatment goal, is a straight line but 'jiggling' contributes significantly to prolonging treatment. The reversal of a tooth movement indicates that the appositional surfaces have to be turned into resorptional surfaces and vice versa. Stopping resorption and starting apposition may not take long, but starting to resorb an osteoid-covered appositional surface may last weeks, as resorption cannot start until mineralization has taken place. The timing of the individual phases of general bone remodeling as described in a study carried out on human biopsies following intravital staining may reflect this relationship [36–38]. Every time an appositional surface has to be turned into a resorptional surface a month of extra treatment time must be added (fig. 7). When performing a treatment analysis the amount of displacement of the individual teeth is rarely more than 5–6 mm, nevertheless the average treatment time does by far exceed that anticipated when the tooth would move directly from point A to point B. The explanation can be found in the use of sliding mechanics and leveling indiscriminately with round wires.

The degrees of freedom when attaching two brackets to a piece of straight wire is as described in the classical paper on the six geometries by Burstone and Koenig [39] will be $6^2 = 36$. When adding 3 teeth together the degrees of freedom will increase to $6^3 = 216$ and so on. It is thus impossible to predict the force system in a statically indeterminate appliance like the continuous arch.

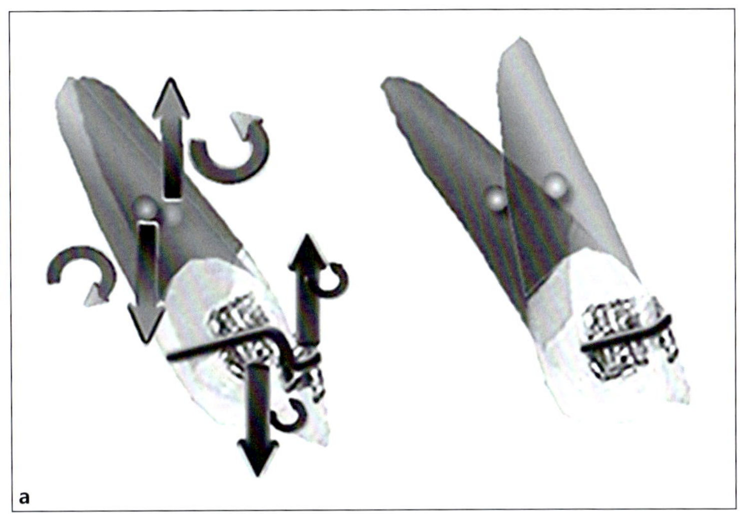

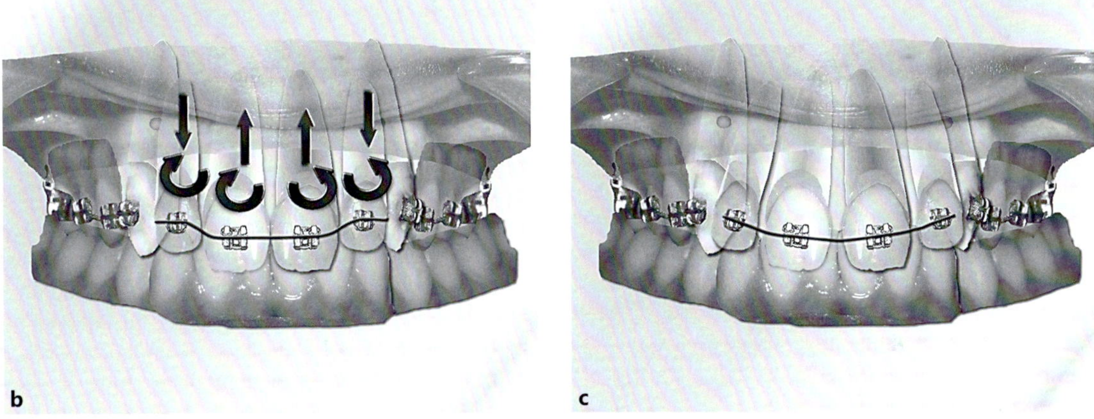

Fig. 6. a To the left, the original problem, i.e. a vertical discrepancy between two incisors. A leveling arch will generate intrusion and lingual root torque on the longer tooth whereas extrusion and lingual root torque will be generated with respect to the short incisor. The situation is reflecting a geometry I according to Burstone and Koenig [39]. **b, c** When the situation is seen from the anterior aspect, a geometry is likewise present generating undesirable side effects with hthe space opening seen in **c**. The correct solution would be to decide whether to intrude the central incisors or to extrude the lateral incisors and not connect the teeth at a different vertical level, and to keep the teeth that are in the correct position: do not connect the good with the bad. Courtesy of G. Fiorelli.

Thanks to growth, the functional matrices and occlusion and the use of intermaxillary elastics an acceptable result is however reached in most cases, although undesirable side effect are not rare and often time consuming to correct.

Several principles should be observed if treatment time should be kept low. 'Jiggling', i.e. changing the direction of the tooth movement should be avoided whenever possible. This implies that oppositely directed nonmeasurable forces acting on one tooth group should be avoided. A class II intermaxillary traction in a patient with need for vertical control of the upper incisors and intrusion built into the upper arch is an example of competing force systems. The connection of the reactive unit, teeth that should stay

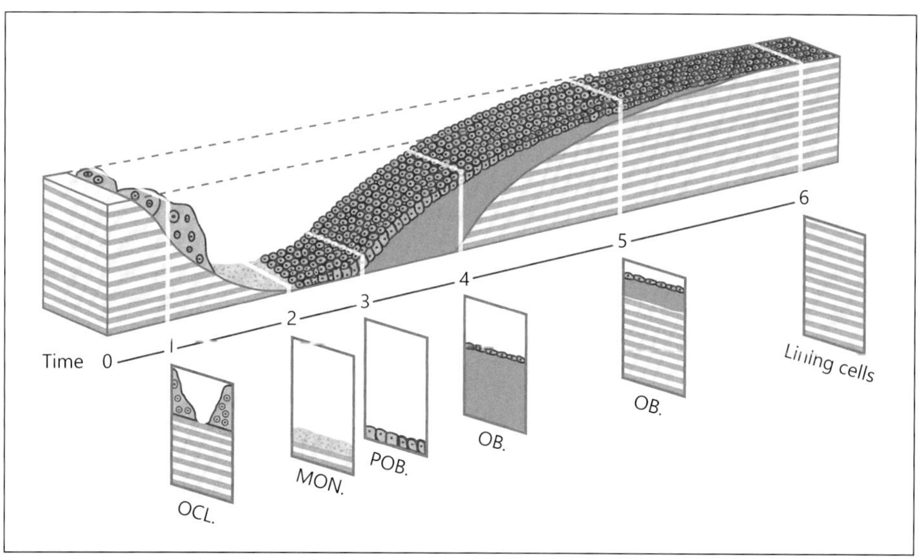

Fig. 7. Graphic illustration of a remodeling unit (ARF), indicating the start with a resorption followed by formation of osteiod that slowly mineralizes. Note the timing of the different sequences. Courtesy of E. Fink Eriksen, 1994.

where they are with the active unit, the teeth to be moved with a continuous archwire will often generate side effects. Root movements before crown movement is recommendable as the turnover is higher in the trabecular bone. Starting with displacement of crowns may render the patients happy, but will in fact prolong the treatment, especially when teeth have to be moved into an extraction space where atrophy has already taken place. Tipping the crowns into the extraction space makes the time for root uprighting even longer than if the space closure is done by translation, or even root movements first.

Avoiding round tripping, 'jiggling', and spending time on tooth movements that cannot take place due to lack of space will help to shorten treatment time. It will prolong treatment, for example, when trying to perform tooth movements with intermaxillary elastics when there is no space.

In a recent book on adult orthodontics [40], the advantages and disadvantages in relation to segmented and custommade segmented appliances were discussed, and it was concluded that in patients where a straight wire would generate side effects a segmented statically determinate appliance would be preferable. The same would be the case in patients with asymmetries and severe periodontal problems with need for true intrusion.

Some advice should be followed if the aim is to shorten treatment time and to control the tooth movements.

(1) Don't connect the good with the bad (citation from Dr. Korn) – in other words decide which teeth to move by defining the treatment goal. Analyze the occlusion carefully and identify whether any units do not have to be displaced. Do not tie these units to the same continuous arch that is connected to units that have to be displaced. Do not start treatment leveling with a round flexible wire of small dimension, if there are any vertical discrepancies because the tooth that is submitted to the extrusive force will also generate a buccal root torque, and the intrusive force will give a lingual root torque. The resulting intra-arch discrepancy in root inclination requires finishing which cannot be obtained by just

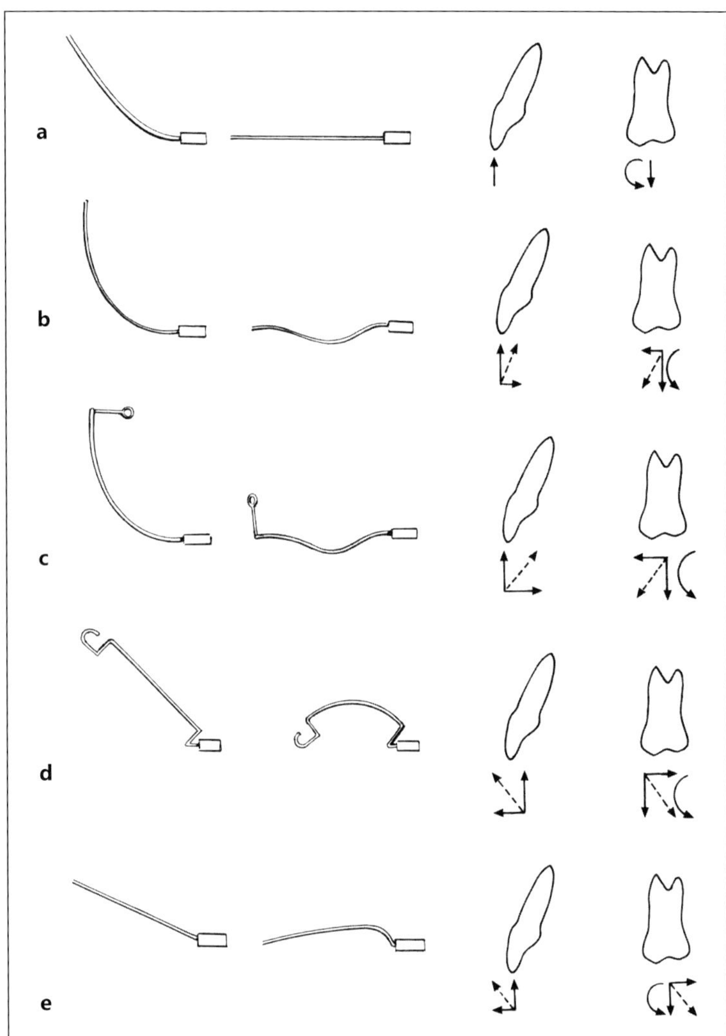

Fig. 8. a–e Illustration of how different configuration of cantilever will influence the direction of the force and thereby the displacement following the insertion of the various cantilevers. Courtesy of G. Fiorelli.

increasing the wire size, as lack of precision of brackets and wires does not allow for sufficient third order control [41].

(2) Make space for the planned tooth movement(s). Start with the correction of the transverse discrepancies. When expansion is desired this should be the first stage of treatment as the widening of the arch is necessary to resolve crowding and problems in other planes of space.

(3) Go as directly to the goal as possible (avoid 'jiggling'). Evaluate whether it is possible to construct an appliance that generates the necessary resultant force directly or whether it may it may be necessary to perform a certain tooth movement in two or even more steps. This could, for example, be necessary in relation to an impacted canine that has to be moved distally in order not to traumatize the incisor roots, then erupted and then finally moved into the arch. However, movement in several directions can often be combined as, for example, intrusion and a sagittal movement performed with a cantilever, the configuration of which will determine the exact direction of the force [42] (fig. 8).

(4) Move roots before crowns. Avoid or reduce the use of appliances that will change the localization of the resultant with respect to the CR of the active unit. This will often be the result of leveling and may lead to extrusion and bite opening which is not always desirable.

Following the guidelines stated above, a statistic of 100 consecutive adult patients in the author's office revealed a median treatment time of 15.6 months ranging from 6 to 33 months. This treatment time corresponds well with what the SureSmile paper claimed and also with the reduction in treatment time recorded following interference with the biological bases through the generation of a RAP phenomenon or a cyclic force delivery.

Combining these approaches with a rational biomechanics, it is possible that the treatment time can be reduced even further. The question regarding cost benefit of the various interventions does, however, still remain to be solved.

References

1 Thilander B: Tissue reactions in orthodontics; in Lee W, Graber RLV Jr (eds): Orthodontics: Current Principles and Techniques. Philadelphia, Elsevier/Mosby, 2012, pp 247–286.
2 Frost HM: Wolff's Law and bone's structural adaptations to mechanical usage: an overview for clinicians. Angle Orthod 1994;64:175–188.
3 Frost HM: Bone's mechanostat: a 2003 update. Anat Rec A Discov Mol Cell Evol Biol 2003;275:1081–1101.
4 Yamasaki K, Shibata Y, Imai S, Tani Y, Shibasaki Y, Fukuhara T: Clinical application of prostaglandin E1 (PGE1) upon orthodontic tooth movement. Am J Orthod 1984;85:508–518.
5 von Bohl M., Maltha JC, von Den Hoff JW, Kuijpers-Jagtman AM: Focal hyalinization during experimental tooth movement in Beagle dogs. Am J Orthod Dentofacial Orthop 2004;125:615–623.
6 von BM, Kuijpers-Jagtman AM: Hyalinization during orthodontic tooth movement: a systematic review on tissue reactions. Eur J Orthod 2009;31:30–36.
7 Davidovitch Z, Finkelson MD, Steigman S, Shanfeld JL, Montgomery PC, Korostoff E: Electric currents, bone remodeling, and orthodontic tooth movement. I. The effect of electric currents on periodontal cyclic nucleotides. Am J Orthod 1980;77:14–32.
8 Davidovitch Z, Finkelson MD, Steigman S, Shanfeld JL, Montgomery PC, Korostoff E: Electric currents, bone remodeling, and orthodontic tooth movement. II. Increase in rate of tooth movement and periodontal cyclic nucleotide levels by combined force and electric current. Am J Orthod 1980;77:33–47.
9 Otter M, Shoenung J, Williams WS: Evidence for different sources of stress-generated potentials in wet and dry bone. J Orthop Res 1985;3:321–324.
10 Melsen B: Biological reaction of alveolar bone to orthodontic tooth movement. Angle Orthod 1999;69:151–158.
11 Cattaneo PM: Orthodontic aspects of bone mechanics and bone remodelling; thesis University of Aarhus, 2003.
12 Cattaneo PM, Dalstra M, Melsen B: The finite element method: a tool to study orthodontic tooth movement. J Dent Res 2005;84:428–433.
13 Dalstra M, Cattaneo PM, Beckmann F, Melsen B: Synchrotron radiation-based micro-tomography of alveolar support tissues. Orthodont Craniofac Res 2006; 9:199–205.
14 Dalstra M, Cattaneo PM, Herzen J, Beckmann F: Visualizing the root-PDL-bone interface using high-resolution microtomography; in Stock SR (ed): Developments in X-Ray Tomography VI. Bellinghamm, SPIE, 2008, pp 70780L1–70780L10.
15 Long H, Pyakurel U, Wang Y, Liao L, Zhou Y, Lai W: Interventions for accelerating orthodontic tooth movement. Angle Orthod 2013;83:164–171.
16 Wilcko MT, Wilcko WM, Murphy KG, Carroll WJ, Ferguson DJ, Miley DD, et al: Full-thickness flap/subepithelial connective tissue grafting with intramarrow penetrations: three case reports of lingual root coverage. Int J Periodontics Restorative Dent 2005;25:561–569.
17 Wilcko MT, Wilcko WM, Pulver JJ, Bissada NF, Bouquot JE: Accelerated osteogenic orthodontics technique: a 1-stage surgically facilitated rapid orthodontic technique with alveolar augmentation. J Oral Maxillofac Surg 2009;67:2149–2159.
18 Kim SJ, Park YG, Kang SG: Effects of Corticision on paradental remodeling in orthodontic tooth movement. Angle Orthod 2009;79:284–291.
19 Kharkar VR, Kotrashetti SM: Transport dentoalveolar distraction osteogenesis-assisted rapid orthodontic canine retraction. Oral Surg Oral Med Oral Pathol Oral Radiol Endod 2010;109:687–693.
20 Melsen B, McNamara JA Jr, Hoenie DC: The effect of bite-blocks with and without repelling magnets studied histomorphometrically in the rhesus monkey (Macaca mulatta). Am J Orthod Dentofacial Orthop 1995;108:500–509.
21 Darendeliler MA, Joho JP: Magnetic activator device II (MAD II) for correction of Class II, division 1 malocclusions. Am J Orthod Dentofacial Orthop 1993;103:223–239.
22 Henao SP, Kusy RP: Evaluation of the frictional resistance of conventional and self-ligating bracket designs using standardized archwires and dental typodonts. Angle Orthod 2004;74:202–211.
23 Kusy RP, Whitley JQ: Friction between different wire-bracket configurations and materials. Semin Orthod 1997;3:166–177.
24 Kusy RP: Influence on binding of third-order torque to second-order angulation. Am J Orthod Dentofacial Orthop 2004;125:726–732.

25 Damon DH: Treatment of the Face with Biocompatible Orthodontics; in Graber TM, Vanarsdall RL, Vig KWL (eds): Orthodontics – Current Principles and Techniques. St. Louis, Elsevier Mosby, 2006, pp 753–832.

26 Scott P, DiBiase AT, Sherriff M, Cobourne MT: Alignment efficiency of Damon3 self-ligating and conventional orthodontic bracket systems: a randomized clinical trial. Am J Orthod Dentofacial Orthop 2008;134:470–478.

27 Andersen KL, Mortensen HT, Pedersen EH, Melsen B: Determination of stress levels and profiles in the periodontal ligament by means of an improved three-dimensional finite element model for various types of orthodontic and natural force systems. J Biomed Eng 1991; 13:293–303.

28 Kau CH: A radiographic analysis of tooth morphology following the use of a novel cyclical force device in orthodontics. Head Face Med 2011;7:14.

29 Nishimura M, Chiba M, Ohashi T, Sato M, Shimizu Y, Igarashi K, et al: Periodontal tissue activation by vibration: intermittent stimulation by resonance vibration accelerates experimental tooth movement in rats. Am J Orthod Dentofacial Orthop 2008;133:572–583.

30 Verna C: The influence of different bone turnover rates on the tissue reactions to orthodontic load; thesis Department of Orthodontics, Aarhus University, 1999.

31 Pilon JJ, Kuijpers-Jagtman AM, Maltha JC: Magnitude of orthodontic forces and rate of bodily tooth movement. An experimental study. Am J Orthod Dentofacial Orthop 1996;110:16–23.

32 Roberts WE, Engen DW, Schneider PM, Hohlt WF: Implant-anchored orthodontics for partially edentulous malocclusions in children and adults. Am J Orthod Dentofacial Orthop 2004;126: 302–304.

33 Guest SS, McNamara JA Jr, Baccetti T, Franchi L: Improving Class II malocclusion as a side-effect of rapid maxillary expansion: a prospective clinical study. Am J Orthod Dentofacial Orthop 2010; 138:582–591.

34 Sachdeva RC, Aranha SL, Egan ME, Gross HT, Sachdeva NS, Currier GF, et al: Treatment time: SureSmile vs conventional. Orthodontics (Chic) 2012;13: 72–85.

35 Hamilton R, Goonewardene MS, Murray K: Comparison of active self-ligating brackets and conventional pre-adjusted brackets. Aust Orthod J 2008;24:102–109.

36 Eriksen EF, Axelrod DW, Melsen F: Bone Histomorphometry. New York, Raven Press, 1994.

37 Eriksen EF: Assessment of erosion depth by lamellar counting. Bone 1993;14: 443–447.

38 Eriksen EF, Gundersen HJ, Melsen F, Mosekilde L: Reconstruction of the formative site in iliac trabecular bone in 20 normal individuals employing a kinetic model for matrix and mineral apposition. Metab Bone Dis Relat Res 1984;5: 243–252.

39 Burstone CJ, Koenig HA: Force systems from an ideal arch. Am J Orthodont 1974;65:270–289.

40 Melsen B, Fiorelli G, Allais D, Mavreas D: Appliance design; in Melsen B (ed): Adult Orthodontics. Chichester, Wiley-Blackwell, 2012, pp 99–131.

41 Eriksen H: Actual vs. theoretical play of 3 conventional and 9 self-ligating bracket systems; thesis submitted for the Speciality in Orthodontics, Department of Orthodontics, Aarhus University, 2011.

42 Dalstra M, Melsen B: Force systems developed by six different cantilever configurations. Clin Orthod Res 1999;2:3–9.

Birte Melsen
Section of Orthodontics, Department of Dentistry, Aarhus University
Vennelyst Boulevard 9
DK–8000 Aarhus C (Denmark)
E-Mail birte@melsen.com

by the lack of function. In dogs, he treated two groups of dogs with an orthodontic appliance that moved both upper and lower second incisors labially for 12–48 h. In half the dogs, their jaws were immobilized by a screen that kept the teeth from contact by the tongue or lips, as well as preventing occlusion. Histologic examination of teeth that were moved as well as control teeth revealed that the first signs of changes were bone formation on the tension side. These initial changes consisted of cell proliferation and formation of osteoid tissue after approximately 36 h. No difference was seen in teeth where there were no functional forces. Human experiments were conducted on the maxillary premolars, presumably moving them before planned extractions. Both loose and attached activators were used to see if pressure from the activator altered the response to force. The activators were adjusted so that control teeth did not contact the plate. Some activators were expanded while others were not.

On the tension side, changes seen with unexpanded loose activators were very minor. No increase in cell number was seen since little or no tension was exerted on the periodontal fibers. Due to the use of the plates, there was a delay in bone formation on the tension side. Signs of resorption were seen in a few instances on the tension side which were thought to be caused by 'daily relapse', where the tooth relapses once the loose plate is removed. The relapse was thought to be due to the contraction of stretched fiber bundles, and Reitan thought this would continue to occur until the periodontal ligament space was sufficiently widened by resorption on the pressure side. Insignificant changes were likewise seen on the pressure side with loose appliances, although there was significant bone resorption with fixed plates at 2, 3 and 4 days.

All the expanded plates demonstrated active bone resorption where there was pressure from expansion. Reitan observed that with no expansion and a loose activator, there was neither resorption nor apposition, presumably due to an insignificant amount of pressure. Thus, Reitan was able to demonstrate that function had no significant influence on the response of teeth to force, but if the force was intermittent, such as with a removable appliance, there would be a delay in bone formation on the tension side due to what he termed 'daily relapse'. This laid the groundwork for additional research into the optimal timing of force.

Other groups also sought to confirm these descriptions with their own methodology. Macapanpan et al. [3] sought to investigate two further questions: what the early tissue changes were, and how the changes were influenced by hormonal or dietary disturbances. They also sought to explore these questions using a rat model. Force was placed on the first and second upper right molars of 35 rats aged 65–70 days using a 3-mm-thick strip of rubber dam stretched between the teeth, with the left side being a control. Animals were sacrificed after 1, 3, 6, 12, 24, 36, 48, 60 and 72 h. Where force was applied, the first molar moved mesially, in contrast to the normal distal drift, and the second and third molars moved distally.

At the cervical level, this movement was noted as little as one hour after placing the rubber dam, although maximum displacement took 12–15 h to occur. The first molar moved significantly more than the other two molars, with a corresponding increased proportion of the degree of widening of the periodontal space, 1.5–1.6 times the second and third molars. The timing of the widening of the periodontal spaces differed between the teeth (fig. 2). Whereas the periodontal ligament space of the first two molars decreased somewhat again after 24 h, the width around the third molar reached its maximum at 12 h but diminished only after 72 h. On the distal side of the first molars, which normally undergo physiologic resorption, there was an arrest of this process within 12 h and a change to apposition 24–36 h after application of force. Increased mitotic activity was also seen on the tension side relative to the control teeth, particularly at 24 and 36 h. This fol-

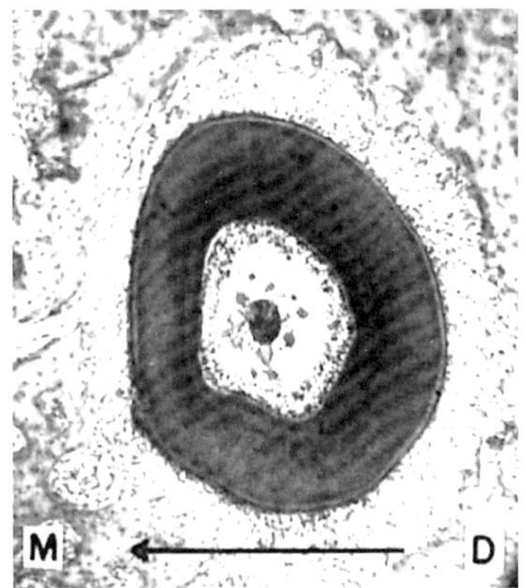

Fig. 2. Difference in the width of the periodontal membranes on the tension (D) and pressure (M) sides of the first molar distolingual root after 1 h of force application. In addition, the periodontal fibers are disorganized and irregular on the pressure side, in contrast to the tension side. From Macapanpan et al. [3].

lowed the maximum displacement of the teeth by 15 to 18 h, and was thought to reflect the initiation of the process of readaptation and repair of the fibers to the altered relationship between the tooth and the bone.

Using this model, the authors specifically looked at the histologic changes under three sets of conditions: (a) when a tooth is moved in the opposite direction as physiologic drift, such as in the first molar; (b) when a tooth is moved in the same direction as physiologic drift, as in the case of the second molar, and (c) when a tooth is moved in the same direction as physiologic drift by means of indirect force, as happens with the third molar. In the first molar, differences between the tension and pressure side were seen as early as one hour after force application: the periodontal fibers on the pressure side were disorganized, frequently with pyknotic nuclei in the fibroblasts. Nuclei in the osteoblasts were compressed, and capillaries were empty. On the tension side, the periodontal fibers and blood vessels were elongated in the direction of tension. Hyalinization was noted beginning at 3 h after force application in the area of greatest pressure. This was comprised of a homog-

enous, cell-free zone with osteoblasts notably absent. Some evidence of undermining resorption in the marrow spaces began to appear. At 12 h, there were no further changes on the pressure side. Undermining resorption had increased in the marrow spaces, and the resorption that usually occurred on the distal surface due to drift had ceased with a decrease in the number of osteoclasts. The process of hyalinization proceeded so that from 24 to 36 h, there was a total loss of fibroblasts in the areas of greatest pressure. At 36 h there was at last evidence of direct resorption on the alveolar side of the first molar, with occasional osteoclasts present, albeit not in areas of hyalinization. Greatly increased mitotic activity was seen on the distal (tension) side of the first molar at this time, with osteoid beginning to be deposited between the periodontal ligament fibers. The authors suggested that this cellular proliferation was part of the process to repair the fibers that had been damaged by the force. From 48 to 72 h, undermining resorption had extended so far on the mesial side that the marrow spaces in some locations had broken through to the periodontal ligament space. In contrast, the control side showed bony apposition on what was normally opposite to the direction of drift. On the distal side, there were increasing young connective tissue cells and osteoid.

In the case of the second molar, the force was applied in the direction of normal drift. As might be expected, the changes seen were similar to the normal situation, but intensified: frontal resorption except adjacent to the hyalinized periodontal membrane, and bone apposition on the tension side. In the third molar, the force was also in the same direction as normal drift, but was indirectly applied. Here, the changes were noted to be similar to those in the second molar but less severe, presumably due to attrition of the force.

In summary, changes seen in the first molar, where the force was applied in the opposite direction to normal drift, some transitional signs were seen, particularly on the distal side of the tooth, where the normal resorption was seen to slow and then cease by approximately 12 h, and then change to apposition by 24–36 h. Increased mitotic activity of the fibroblasts was also seen on the tension side which was 3–4 times that on the control side. The authors concluded that fibroblasts were an important contributor to the response to force, in addition to osteoclasts and osteoblasts.

In that same year, Waldo and Rothblatt [4] offered their own technique for studying tooth movement in rats which corroborated Macapanpan's. They also proposed that small mammals would be easier to use than the baboons that Oppenheim used. In addition, they suggested that the genetic variability in rats could be much more easily controlled. Their technique involved stretching strips of an intermaxillary elastic, 8 mm in thickness between the first and second maxillary molars of a rat. No additional interventions took place, and the animals were sacrificed after times ranging from 24 h to 1 week. Baseline observations with no tooth movement revealed random trabeculation of bone with uniform width of the periodontal membrane. After 24 h, some response, though minimal, was observed: the width of the periodontal membrane was decreased in areas of pressure accompanied by a localized vasoconstriction. The opposite was seen in areas of tension. After three days, the tissue response was near its maximum, which often included hemorrhage and undermining resorption. The periodontal membrane was again compressed in the area of pressure. Changes were also seen in the opposing quadrant, presumably due to altered occlusion resulting from slight tipping of the molar. These changes represented adaptation to the altered maxillary occlusion, so that normal occlusal contacts were re-established. Histologic examination of the bone at this time period shows bony resorption and remodeling on the pressure side with large numbers of multinucleated osteoclasts. Undermining resorption was noted in areas where the periodontal membrane was completely or nearly completely compressed and in areas of hemorrhage.

The response at 5 days was more marked than after 3 days, and a similar response was noted between the second and third molars, which did not have the elastic placed but nonetheless experienced the force from the second molar. For the first time, thin streamers of new bone are seen on the tension side, while Howship's lacunae are seen on the pressure side demonstrating osteoclastic activity. Another demonstration of the response to pressure was occasionally seen in the form of external root resorption. Waldo and Rothblatt hypothesized that this was part of a normal spectrum of response to excessive force. Reaction to the force was again noted in the lower arch, demonstrating tooth movement in the lower arch in reaction to opposing dental movement. These reactions included bony deposition in the presumptive area of tension and narrowing of the periodontal membrane and bony resorption in areas of pressure. In comparing this study to Macapanpan's, Waldo and Rothblatt [3] used a much thicker elastic material to apply the force (0.8 vs. 0.3 mm). The greater severity of response seen by Waldo and Rothblatt is likely due to this difference.

Zaki and Van Huysen [5] applied this technique to 24 rats, placing the rubber between the maxillary first and second molars. This resulted in the first molar tipping mesially and the second molar tipping distally. Six rats were sacrificed at 6 h, 6 at 12 h, 6 at 24 h, and 6 at 72 h. In each group, sections were made in each of the three planes of space for evaluation of cellular changes. After 6 h, there was narrowing of the periodontal ligament space on the mesial or pressure side of the root in the cervical third. The fibers were indistinct with fewer nuclei within the fibroblasts. Furthermore, the nuclei were pyknotic, leading the authors to conclude that the process of hyalinization was beginning. These changes were also seen on the mesial aspect of the distal root, which nearly contacted the interradicular bone. In addition, there was osteoclastic resorption within the medullary spaces of adjacent bone, signifying the beginning of undermining resorption. On the distal aspect of all roots, as well as the mesial aspect of the distally-tipped second molar, stretching of the PDL fibers was noted. The nuclei of these fibroblasts were elongated in the direction of the tension.

At 12 h, these changes were more definite. On the pressure sides of the molar roots, distinct hyalinization was observed. Fibroblasts continued to be fewer in number than on the tension side, with pyknotic nuclei. However, in the medullary spaces adjoining the osteoclastic alveolar ridge resorption, osteoblasts were now seen, in contrast to the earlier observation of osteoclasts. On the tension side, the fibroblasts were numerous and exhibited plump nuclei with blood vessels interspersed that had ovoid lumina.

At 24 h, the pressure sides of the roots still showed significant compression of the PDL with varying degrees of hyalinization. The tension side had increased cellular proliferation at the alveolar bone surface, and a layer of osteoid was observed at the ends of the fibroblasts. Osteoblasts were seen atop this layer of osteoid.

At 72 h, the surface of the bone on the pressure side was covered with many osteoclasts. Some blood vessels were thrombosed. The PDL fibers were compressed and disorganized, but connective cell proliferation was also seen.

Zaki and Van Huysen [5] noted that their results agreed with those of Sandstedt regarding the speed of the response to force, with significant changes observed after only 6 h. They noted, however, that bone is constantly remodeling and changes due to this normal process must be differentiated from those due to external force application. Additionally, they observed the total lack of inflammatory changes accompanying the cellular response to force. This may be due to the fact that the rubber material used in Zaki and Van Huysen's study was only 0.14 mm thick, as opposed to the previous studies, where materials 2–5 times thicker were used.

Tayer et al. [6] used dogs in their 1968 investigation of the role of proliferation of osteoclasts and osteoblasts during tooth movement. They injected tritiated thymidine into a dog's carotid artery 28 days following the initiation of orthodontic tooth movement using 140 g of force. Six hours later, they sacrificed the dog and processed alternate sections of the jaws for hematoxylin and eosin staining and autoradiographic analysis. Routine histologic analysis revealed findings similar to those described above, with a disorganized PDL and hyaline degeneration on the pressure side and bone apposition with rear bone resorption on the tension side that served to maintain the width of the PDL. However, there was significant labeling of the nuclei of both osteoclasts and osteoblasts in both the areas of pressure and tension. The authors concluded that the presence of cell labeling in areas of hyalinization suggested that these cells originated at least in part from local precursor cell, possibly undifferentiated mesenchymal cells. They proposed that this could represent a repair process, similar to that proposed by Macapanpan et al. [3]. They concluded by stating that cellular proliferation in the periodontal ligament in response to orthodontic force may be dependent upon the magnitude of the force.

Gianelly [7] continued to investigate the response to tooth movement in his 1969 paper evaluating the changes in vascularity in the PDL following force application. He sought to determine the exact relationship between the amount of force, vascular patency, and type of resorption. Gianelly noted that the two kinds of bone resorption – frontal and undermining – were related to the integrity of the PDL, which correspondingly depended upon the vascular supply. Forces which were lighter did not occlude or damage the local blood vessels, and resorption on the surface of the bone resulted. On the other hand, heavier forces obliterated the vascular supply so that resorption and remodeling had to be initiated in the neighboring medullary spaces and gradually reach the area of direct pressure. In a series of two experiments, Gianelly used elastics forced between the maxillary canines and incisors of dogs. These were placed on the left side only so that the right side served as a control. Carbon black suspension was infused into the carotid arteries of each animal shortly before sacrifice. In the first experiment, the infusion and sacrifice were carried out 10 min after force application, whereas in the second, the force application was maintained for 7 days before infusion and sacrifice. Elastics of varying forces were used in each experiment. Results from immediate sacrifice showed that application of 50 g of force resulted in slightly diminished vascularity in the pressure area as compared to the control area. Application of 100 g showed additional diminution of vascularity, while 150 g resulted in total occlusion of the blood vessels. When the force was maintained for 7 days, application of 75 g showed very little changes in the amount of vascularity, with frontal resorption carried out. Both frontal and undermining resorption resulted from application of 125 g of force. Gianelly concluded that changes in the vasculature after applying orthodontic force may determine the pattern of bone resorption. He referred to Bien's theory of hydrostatic damping of the vasculature and hypothesized that if the vessels were obliterated by excessive force, they could not function as damping agents and tooth movement could not proceed by normal means.

A later paper by Reitan [8] further investigated the tissue reaction to force with varying amounts of force, direction of force, and the age of the patient. Comparison of tissues from a 12-year-old patient with those of someone in their 30s revealed fewer cells evident in the periodontal ligament, with no osteoblasts and little osteoid tissue. Reitan noted that this would mean a delay in the time required for cell proliferation that is needed to lay down bone: 8 days in an adult compared with the usual 1–2 days in the adolescent. Reitan recommended applying light forces during the initial stages of tooth movement in order to avoid the hyalinized areas that were noted on the pressure side. This cell-free layer is caused by forces exceeding the capacity of the alveolus to resorb, resulting in necrosis in the membrane cells. As a result, an indirect resorption process must be initiated, leading to a lag time of up to 2 weeks in duration before tooth movement can occur.

Reitan went on to describe the different types of force: continuous, intermittent, and interrupted. Reitan particularly mentioned interrupted forces as a situation where an activated archwire gradually becomes less active as the tooth moves. While a hyalinized area may be created on the pressure side, it will be removed by resorption, and the force will decrease rapidly as the tooth moves, thereby 'interrupting' the force. He contrasted this with intermittent force such as was used in removable appliances, where the resorption process is discontinued as the appliance is removed. These intermittent forces were observed to be compatible with favorable nutritional conditions with increased blood circulation, an increased number of cells, and thereby direct resorption of bone. However, there was significant variation in individual response. Reitan concluded that functional intermittent forces of 70–100 g could cause formation of cell-free (hyalinized) areas, but these were less extensive and of shorter duration than with continuous forces.

Reitan proceeded to compare the tissue reaction found in a tipping movement with that found in bodily movement. Because the tooth acts as a lever in a tipping movement, the crestal force will always be greater with a tipping movement than with a bodily movement. This explains why hyalinized areas are less frequently found in bodily movement. Reitan then applied these concepts to specific methods of tooth movement, pointing out that if a sectional wire places too much force on an isolated tooth, it will not move because hyalinization will occur, and the anchor teeth will move instead. He recommended using a continuous wire in these situations so that the force could be shared by the anterior teeth.

Applications of these concepts need to take tooth size into account. Because of differences in the size of tooth roots, more absolute force will be required to move some teeth to maintain the optimal range of force per square millimeter of tooth surface. Reitan recommended 150–250 g for a maxillary canine, 100–200 g for mandibular canines, and less for premolars. Reitan also discussed the use of torque. He pointed out that torquing forces will be least strong at the apical area, and that a force at the apex of 130 g would produce direct bone resorption without any hyalinized areas.

In summary, Reitan described how to achieve tooth movement that minimized the amount of hyalinization and maximized direct bone resorption. Depending on the tooth, direction and type of movement, this force varied considerably: from 250 g for bodily movement of canines to 25 g to extrude a single incisor.

In 1972, Buck and Church [9] reported on a study they had carried out to investigate how the periodontal ligament responded to a light force with regards to the establishment of a cell-free zone. They had placed a fixed palatal appliance in 12 adolescents aged 11–15 years who were treatment planned for extraction of the maxillary first bicuspids. The appliance tipped the bicuspids buccally with fingersprings using a force of 70 ± 7 g. After 7, 14, 21 or 28 days, the teeth were extracted along with 5 mm of buccal bone. After fixation, decalcification, and paraffin embedding of the root and bone, 7-μm transverse sections were cut and stained for histologic examination. The narrowest width of the PDL space was measured, and the degree of cellular loss within the PDL space and the distance from the alveolar crest were recorded.

At 7 days, all specimens showed PDL compression of an average of 64 μm. All specimens showed some portion of the PDL that was cellfree. The extent of this area was an average of 1.15 mm in height, with predominance toward the alveolar crest. All samples had undermining resorption. At the more apical areas, there was frontal resorption and less cell-free area. New bone proliferation was noted in all but one of the sam-

ples. By 14 days, there was only a very localized cell-free area and very limited compression of the PDL. Immature bone was seen in all samples. After 21 days, there was more pronounced individual variation. A widened PDL space was found, with very little osteoclastic activity. Osteoblastic activity predominated, with reorganization of the PDL. This reorganization was the main feature seen at 28 days. Buck and Church concluded that there was no significant lag phase with the level of force used, and frontal resorption was possible. However, cell-free areas did exist, particularly at seven days. They admitted that the effect of reactivation of these types of forces was unknown.

All these observations and experiments were interpreted through the framework of the pressure-tension model, whereby the two sides of the tooth seemed to respond to the pressure as if in isolation from one another. For example, one of the introductory sentences in Tayer's paper describes, 'A force applied to a tooth creates areas of pressure and tension'. This simplistic model satisfied many clinicians for many years.

However, a second major theory of how a tooth responds to force was being concurrently investigated. In 1938, Stuteville [10] had proposed a hydraulic system of tooth movement. Stuteville observed that the peridental membrane contained blood vessels from three sources: from the tooth apex, through the walls of the alveolus, and over the crest of the alveolus. The blood in this vasculature as well as lymph and intercellular fluid has intrinsic pressure, and when the tooth has no forces acting on it, the peridental membrane is relaxed. However, when extrinsic pressure acts upon the tooth, the hydraulic pressure increases immediately, and blood is forced out of the vessels through the cribriform plate in the alveolar wall as the tooth moves in the direction of the force. When the force is released, the tooth returns to its resting position and the vessels fill again with blood. During force application, the peridental fibers, which have no elasticity, serve to limit the movement of the tooth. No permanent changes occur with forces of mastication, when the force only lasts for a short period of time. When forces are prolonged; however, the bony surface of the alveolus may resorb or lay down more bone to maintain a constant width of the peridental membrane. Additionally, the membrane may become necrotic or tear with prolonged or extreme force.

In 1966, Bien [11] explained his hypothesis of hydrodynamic damping of tooth movement. He described three 'distinct but interacting' fluid systems that participated in the response of the tooth to force: first, the vascular system in the blood and lymphatic vessels; second, the system of the periodontal membrane fibers; and third, the interstitial fluid that exists among all the cells, bone, tooth, vessels, and fibers. Bien measured the reaction to an intrusive force on a rat incisor, both with alive and dead rats. By way of complex measurements and calculations, Bien arrived at the 'Reynolds number', which is the ratio of inertial forces to viscous forces, and the spring constant, used to evaluate the damping capacity of the system under different loads. He observed both an intrusive movement and a return movement as the force was removed. The difference in these movements was significant and indicated the source of damping. Bien interpreted this information to explain what happens when a tooth is intruded. During the intrusive force application, extracellular fluids are squeezed into the marrow space from the periodontal space. Once these fluids are exhausted, the periodontal fibers tighten and slow the movement of the tooth. As the fibers tighten, they also constrict the small blood vessels, further impeding blood flow. At this point, fluid must filter through the vessel walls to escape, but there is a significant increase in pressure in the blood vessels. Figures obtained from dead rats represented the contribution of extracellular fluid flow, since fluids are not replenished in the dead animal. The figures were different but still within the same order of magnitude, demonstrating that the resistance to force is predominantly due to viscous forces. Although it is unclear how these observations dovetail with the traditional, cellular responses to force using the 'pressure-tension' theory, it is clear that fluids, fluid flow, and resistance to movement by fluids and fibers must be considered in elucidating the complete mechanism of response to force including tooth movement.

Baumrind [12] expanded on this theory in his 1969 article by testing whether the traditional pressure-tension theory accounted for all of the observations seen during tooth movement. He reported on studies that investigated the reaction in the PDL as measured by metabolic activity, rate of cell replication, and rate of fiber synthesis using tritiated amino acids as markers for activity. They also sought to investigate dimensional changes in the PDL. Baumrind used Waldo's method of experimental tooth movement in a rat model to examine these reactions. Measurements were made during the first 72 h following placement of the rubber dam material unilaterally in 33 rats. The unilateral nature of the method allowed a three-way comparison between the treated side, untreated side, and an untreated animal.

Preliminary observations revealed that metabolic changes on the tension and pressure sides of the tooth always occurred in the same direction, with cell replication rates increasing and collagen synthesis decreasing on both sides. This led Baumrind to focus on dimensional changes on the mesial (pressure) and distal (tension) aspects of the first molar, both of which were remote from the force application and any possible local trauma. The area on the distal aspect studied was the most occlusal microscope field below the furcation, while the area on the mesial aspect was the microscope field that included the alveolar crest as its occlusal most point. When the elastic band was placed interproximally, the interproximal space increased by an average of 335 µm. However, the distance between the apices of the teeth only increased an average of 14 µm, implying a significant tipping movement of the teeth. However, in the pressure region, the reduction of width of the PDL averaged only 15 μm, while on the tension side, there was an average increase of only 4 μm. Baumrind pointed out that the discrepancy between movement of the tooth crowns was ten times larger than the average reduction in PDL width on the pressure side. He felt that this could only be accounted for by some bending of the alveolar bone, and further hypothesized that this deflection of the bone was being produced by forces lower than what was required for reduction in the width of the PDL.

Baumrind goes on to suggest that, in accordance with Pascal's Law, any force delivered to the periodontal ligament will be transmitted equally to all areas of the PDL. This equalization of pressure will occur regardless of any deflection of the bone. Thus, if any fluids are squeezed out of the PDL, they would be squeezed out in all areas. He went on to propose a comprehensive theory of his own: when orthodontic forces are placed, they are transmitted equally to all the tissues in the area: bone, tooth, and PDL. Each type of material will deform to some extent. As part of the response to deformation, the bone will re-model through tissue turnover. Baumrind also believed that the PDL changed in response, but that this response was too small to be the only response. He points out that this hypothesis answers many questions that are not readily explained by the pressure-tension theory: why en masse closure is relatively slow, why anterior teeth can frequently move so quickly, and why teeth can move so quickly into an extraction site.

Despite these observations and publications, many major textbooks continue to refer to the process of tooth movement as one of resorption on the pressure side and deposition on the tension side. It is clear that both the pressure-tension and fluid flow concepts have merit, and it is likely that the truth contains elements of both. However, it is also clear that considerable work needs to be done to ascertain the details. The following papers will explore modern aspects of tooth movement and what recent research has uncovered. It is hoped that future research will build on these contemporary efforts so that tooth movement can be managed and controlled for the benefit of the patient.

References

1 Oppenheim A: Tissue changes particularly of bone, incident to tooth movement. Am Orthod 1911–2;3:57–67, 113–132.
2 Reitan K: The tissue reaction as related to the functional factor. Trans Eur Orthod Soc 1951;27:123–136.
3 Macapanpan LC, Weinmann JP, Brodie AG: Early tissue changes following tooth movement in rats. Angle Orthod 1954; 24:79–95.
4 Waldo CM, Rothblatt JM: Histologic response to tooth movement in the laboratory rat. J Dent Res 1954;33:481–486.
5 Zaki AE, van Huysen G: Histology of the periodontium following tooth movement. J Dent Res 1963;42:1373–1379.
6 Tayer BH, Gianelly AA, Ruben MP: Visualization of cellular dynamics associated with orthodontic tooth movement. Am J Orthod 1968;54:515–520.
7 Gianelly AA: Force-induced changes in the vascularity of the periodontal ligament. Am J Orthod 1969;55:5–11.
8 Reitan K: Some factors determining the evaluation of forces in orthodontics. Am J Orthod 1957;43:32–45.
9 Buck DL, Church DH: A histologic study of tooth movement. Am J Orthod 1972; 62:507–516.
10 Stuteville OH: A summary review of tissue changes incident to tooth movement. Angle Orthod 1938;8:1–20.
11 Bien SM: Hydrodynamic damping of tooth movement. J Dent Res 1966;45: 907–914.
12 Baumrind S: A reconsideration of the propriety of the 'pressure-tension' hypothesis. Am J Orthod 1969;55:12–22.

Leslie A. Will, DMD, MSD
Department of Orthodontics and Dentofacial Orthopedics
Boston University Goldman School of Dental Medicine
100 East Newton Street, Room 104
Boston, MA 02118 (USA)
E-Mail willla@bu.edu

Kantarci A, Will L, Yen S (eds): Tooth Movement. Front Oral Biol. Basel, Karger, 2016, vol 18, pp 56–63
DOI: 10.1159/000353098

Stability and Retention

Leslie A. Will

Department of Orthodontics and Dentofacial Orthopedics, Boston University Goldman School of Dental Medicine,
Boston, Mass., USA

Abstract

Stability of tooth position in the broader sense considers all the forces that may act on the tooth. Reitan reported that significant forces remained in the periodontium after tooth movement, and he carried out research that demonstrated residual stretching of the crestal periodontal fibers more than 7 months after tooth movement. Brain demonstrated that severing the fibers reduced the relapse in tooth position in dogs. Edwards published a series of papers exploring the effects of surgical transection of the gingival fibers on tooth stability, recommending that circumferential fiberotomy be performed in order to increase posttreatment tooth stability. Other researchers have suggested ways to increase the stability of the incisors, which are typically most prone to relapse. Peck and Peck recommended that interproximal reduction be done to broaden the contact point. Boese also recommended interproximal reduction as part of a four-pronged approach to retention.

Stability of tooth position can be considered in several different contexts. To researchers, maintenance of tooth position implies analysis and balance of the forces acting on a tooth. It is commonly recognized that a tooth will move if force is placed upon it. During treatment, the force is intentionally placed using the elastic force of metal wires and springs or perhaps elastomers. These forces supercede those forces that already exist in the environment of each tooth: masticatory forces, forces from the surrounding soft tissues such as the tongue, lips, and cheeks, and even forces created by parafunctional habits, including digit sucking and bruxing. However, after orthodontic treatment, these background forces come to the fore once again and, if not in balance with respect to the tooth's new position, can lead to tooth movement that is interpreted as relapse.

Because it is difficult to quantify these forces, it is difficult to predict when an orthodontically treated tooth may relapse. Many studies have been carried out to identify predictive factors for instability and many treatment situations where posttreatment relapse is often observed. Incisor irregularity is often taken as the definition of relapse since it is the most easily detected. In addition, any form of arch expansion, such as widening of the dental arch, proclination of incisors, and increase in the intercanine distance is also associated with instability.

Besides looking at orthodontic tooth movement that may lead to relapse, most orthodontic

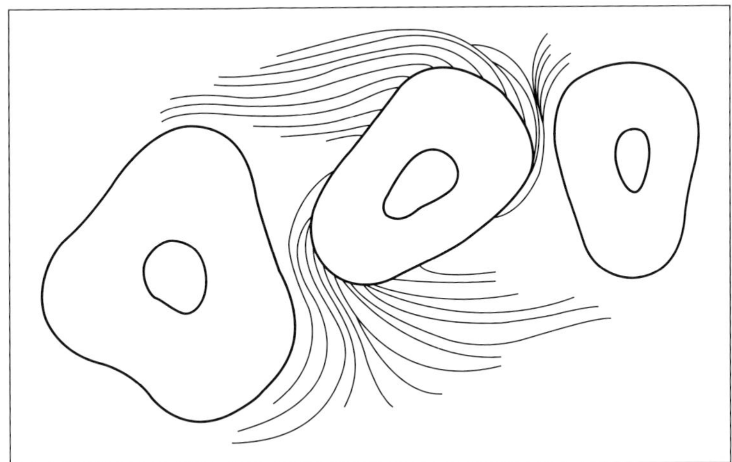

Fig. 1. The arrangement of free gingival fibers following rotation of the teeth. From Reitan [1, fig 5, p 107].

textbooks deal with stability from a clinical, procedural point of view and describe which retainers are used with which protocol. It seems that the more important discussion is the one regarding how to place teeth in a position that is more stable. To do this, the evidence regarding which factors influence the position of a tooth after treatment, i.e. stability, must be examined.

There is little consensus regarding the precise factors governing stability, but the incontrovertible evidence is that if force is placed on a tooth, it will move, and a variety of forces can be acting on the tooth even after orthodontic treatment. These forces include forces from the periodontium, both the supracrestal fibers and the periodontal ligament, forces of occlusion, forces from soft tissue outside the periodontium, muscle forces, and forces from the dentition.

In 1959, Reitan [1] reported that significant forces remained in the periodontium after tooth movement. He rotated the second upper incisor in dogs over 8–12 weeks, and retained the rotated tooth for 15–232 days. The fibers supporting the teeth were shown to stretch and displace during tooth movement, and then tended to rearrange over time and become realigned perpendicular to the surface of the tooth. Histologic examination of the fibers at the apical, middle, and crestal re-

gions showed great differences in the degrees of rearrangement of the fibers after varying amounts of retention (fig. 1). Of the six teeth examined, two never rearranged at any level following a short retention period of 15 days. Conversely, at the apical region, there was fairly good rearrangement of the fibers by 28 days, with complete rearrangement by 83 days of retention. At the middle region, complete rearrangement took slightly longer, while at the crestal region, the fibers remained stretched in accordance with the direction of rotation even after 232 days – more than 7 months. This was noted to be particularly true of the fiber bundles on the labial and lingual surfaces of the root.

The bone was also noted to respond and rearrange in response to the force, with new bone laid down along stretched fiber bundles. Once again, more rapid realignment was seen in the apical region, with significant rearrangement taking place by 57 days but essentially complete realignment by 147 days. The middle region again was comparatively slightly slower to demonstrate realignment, with complete realignment noted only after 232 days. At the crestal area, no rearrangement was seen until 57 days, and even at the longest observation period the response was modest.

Kantarci A, Will L, Yen S (eds): Tooth Movement. Front Oral Biol. Basel, Karger, 2016, vol 18, pp 64–74
DOI: 10.1159/000351900

Neurologic Regulation and Orthodontic Tooth Movement

Stephanos Kyrkanides · Hechang Huang · Richard D. Faber

Department of Orthodontics and Pediatric Dentistry, School of Dental Medicine, Stony Brook University, Stony Brook, N.Y., USA

Abstract

Pain and discomfort are prevalent symptoms among the vast majority of patients with fixed orthodontic appliances and is the most disliked aspect of treatment. The periodontium is a highly innervated structure that also provides the necessary trophic factors, such as nerve growth factor, which promote neuronal survival, maintenance and axonal growth, via interaction with specific nerve surface receptors, such as TrkA. Various types of nerves are found in the periodontium, including thinly myelinated and unmyelinated sensory fibers that express the neuropeptides substance P and calcitonin gene-related peptide among others. Tooth movement activates peripheral sensory nerve endings, which transmit painful signals to the brain after being processed at the trigeminal spinal nucleus, resulting in local expression of pain related genes, such as c-Fos. Concurrently, an attendant inflammatory process is detected in the trigeminal spinal nucleus, including activation of astrocytes, microglia and neurons. This complex neurologic reaction to tooth movement mediates orthodontic pain and also serves a source of neurogenic inflammation exhibited in the trigeminal spinal nucleus and the periodontium. Activated periodontal sensory fibers release neuropeptides in the periodontal environment, which in turn induce a local inflammatory cascade aiding in alveolar bone turnover and tooth movement per se. Control of pain with nonsteroidal anti-inflammatory drugs and other prescription or over-the-counter pain killers effectively reduce this neurologic reaction and alleviate the attendant pain, but also reduce the neurogenic inflammatory component of orthodontic tooth movement causing a slowdown in bone turnover and consequently delaying orthodontic treatment.
© 2016 S. Karger AG, Basel

Orthodontic Pain

Patient discomfort and/or pain is quite prevalent among orthodontic patients with fixed appliances, ranging from 91 to 95% among different patient populations [1–3], and is the most disliked aspect of orthodontic treatment [4]. Most patients reported feeling discomfort or pain within 4 h after initial placement of separators or arch wires which peaks at 24 h and is gradually alleviated in 5–7 days [3, 5–8], while in a small portion of patients the pain can last more than 4 weeks [6]. The pain and discomfort is more pronounced in the anterior than in the posterior region [3, 7, 9], and more pronounced in the mandibular than in the maxillary arch [10]. The pain caused by orthodontic treatment has a minor to moderate impact on patients' daily and social life [3], but at its peak leads to being awakened at night in about 20% of patients [1, 3] and to switching to a softer diet in about 60% of patients [3]. Pain and discomfort induced by orthodontic treatment is among the major fears before orthodontic treatment [4] and a leading cause of discontinuing treatment [5, 11, 12]. The degree of initial anterior and posterior crowding makes no difference in the overall discomfort and pain experience [13]. Two independent studies revealed that heavier forces caused more intense initial pain compared to lighter forces [14, 15]. The degree of pain may also be affected by the type of orthodontic appliance employed. It has been shown that fixed appliances can cause higher intensity of pain compared to removable appliances [16, 17], while others report no differences between fixed and removable orthodontic appliances [12]. When the same size, the superelastic NiTi archwire causes less initial pain compared to conventional NiTi archwire during the first 10 h after archwire placement [10], and thermoelastic NiTi archwire causes less initial pain compared to superelastic NiTi archwire at days 2, 3 and 4 after archwire placement [18]. On the other hand, the percentage of patients experiencing pain is not significantly different between patients receiving 0.014 and 0.016 inch NiTi arch wires used in the initial alignment of teeth [9]. With self-ligating brackets, Damon3® brackets do not appear to affect the perception of pain and discomfort compared to conventional brackets during the first week of treatment [19]. SmartClip® brackets showed similar effects during the first week of treatment, but cause significantly more pain during arch wire insertion and removal [20]. Damon® SL-II brackets reportedly induce a lower level of pain compared to conventional brackets during the first week of treatment, but do not reduce usage of analgesics by patients [21]. Wu et al. [22] found that the overall level of pain was not significantly different between patients treated with labial or lingual fixed orthodontic appliances, but patients treated with labial appliances reported a higher intensity of pain in the lips and cheeks, while those treated with lingual appliance reported a higher intensity of pain in the tongue. In addition to routine fixed orthodontic appliances, some other appliances also cause pain and discomfort during treatment, including rapid maxillary expander [23], headgear [24], Herbst appliance [25] and chin cup [26].

The perception of pain by orthodontic patients is subjective and shows considerable individual variations. Patient's age, gender, cultural environment and emotional/cognitive factors may influence perception of pain. The level of perceived pain was higher in adult orthodontic patients (older than 16 years) than in adolescents [5, 6, 27]. In contrast with these findings, Scheurer et al. [3] discovered that the frequency of pain was the highest in patients of 13–16 years, followed by those older age than 16 and 10–13 years. However, Ngan et al. [7] found that there was no difference between patients of younger or older than 16 years in perception of pain after insertion of separators and initial arch wires. The inconsistency may be due to different study designs. As for the influence of gender, two studies showed that more females reported pain than males [1, 3], while other surveys showed that there was no difference in pain between the sexes [6, 7, 9, 10]. The discrepancy may be due to differences in population (age group and culture) or survey methods. Sociocultural factors may also affect responses to pain. Ethnicity, psychology and culture affect experimental pain responses [28]. Different attitudes and behaviors to pain expected by different cultures (e.g. stoic vs. demonstrative)

Fig. 1. PGP 9.5 expressing nerve fibers in the periodontium. **a** Parasagittal histology section of a mouse maxilla stained by HE showing upper molars. **b** PGP 9.5 immunofluorescence depicting nerve fibers located within the periodontal ligament (green) contrasted by nuclear Hoechst counterstain (blue).

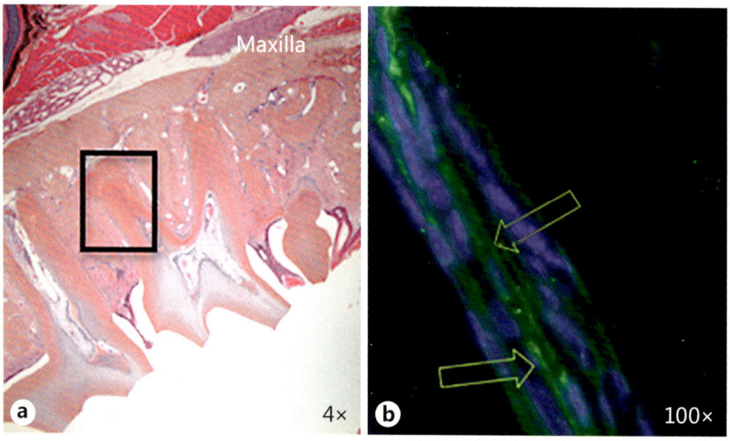

may affect an individual's perception and reporting of pain [29, 30]. However, to date there is no study on the effects of cultural factors on response of pain to orthodontic treatment. Emotional factors, such as anxieties and fears, are not uncommon among people receiving orthodontic treatment. It was demonstrated that anxiety levels are positively associated with reports of pain [31], and anxiety may lower the pain threshold and cause perception of nonpainful stimuli as painful [32]. Therefore, the perception of pain may be influenced by the emotional status of patients. Cognitive factors, including motivation, expectations, beliefs, attention/distraction and feeling of control may also affect an individual's perception of pain [29].

Induction of Orthodontic Pain

The periodontium is richly innervated by sensory fibers that have either mechanoreceptors or nociceptors responsible to perceive mechanical pressure or pain, respectively, as well as supplied by autonomic fibers that are responsible to regulate blood flow in the periodontium [33–38]. Immunohistofluorescent staining of protein gene product (PGP) 9.5, a neural-specific marker, reveals abundant existence of neural fibers in the peri-

odontium (fig. 1), providing an anatomical basis for the close interactions of neural and other kinds of tissues during orthodontic tooth movement.

Neurotrophins, namely neuronal growth factor (NGF) are diffusible micro-environmental factors critical to neuronal survival, maintenance and axonal growth [39, 40]. We find that in the periodontium, NGF is expressed by alveolar bone and periodontal ligament cells under naïve conditions (fig. 2). In addition to its neurotrophic function, NGF mediates inflammatory pain during orthodontic treatment [41] that will be described with more detail in a section below.

NGF binds with high affinity to its cell membrane tyrosine kinase (Trk) A receptor, which is abundantly expressed by neural fibers in the periodontal ligament (PDL) under resting conditions (fig. 3). Binding to TrkA is crucial for the neurotrophic function of NGF as demonstrated by mice lacking TrkA expression [42]. NGF production is stimulated by inflammatory factors such as tumor necrosis factor-α and other cytokines. Following internalization, the NGF-TrkA complex is transported to the primary sensory neuron body, where it upregulates the expression of substance P (SP) and calcitonin gene-related peptide (CGRP), which are potent neuropeptides causing

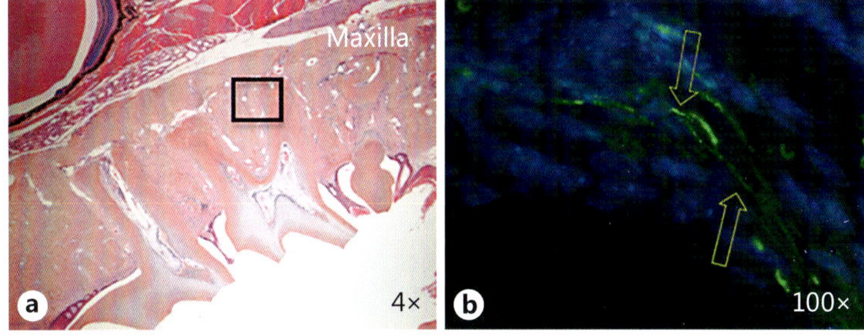

Fig. 2. The neurotrophin NGF is expressed in the periodontium. The NGF promotes neuronal survival, maintenance and axonal growth in the periodontium. **a** Parasagittal histology section of a mouse maxilla stained by HE showing upper molars. **b** NGF immunofluorescence depicting neurotrophin expression by osteocytes in the alveolar bone as well as a multitude of cells in the periodontal ligament (green) contrasted by nuclear Hoechst counterstain (blue).

Fig. 3. TrkA is expressed on nerve fibers in the periodontium. The tyrosine receptor kinase A (TrkA) is a cell surface receptor with high affinity for the NGF expressed by the periodontium. **a** Parasagittal histology section of a mouse maxilla stained by H&E showing upper molars. **b** TrkA–expressing nerve fibers localized in the periodontal ligament (green) contrasted by nuclear Hoechst counterstain (blue).

neurogenic inflammation [43, 44]. Orthodontic tooth movement can also increase production of NGF as well as TrkA in the PDL [45].

Pain from orthodontic tooth movement results from the activation of nociceptive fibers in the periodontium, such as small diameter unmyelinated (C fibers) and thinly myelinated nerve (Aδ) fibers [44], during tooth movement. These nociceptive nerve fibers are characterized by the expression of neuropeptides such as SP and CGRP, the expression of which is often colocalized [46]. We find such SP-positive nerve fibers proximal to the apex of teeth (fig. 4).

The physiological mechanism of pain during orthodontic tooth movement is complex. Local ischemia from compression of blood vessels in the PDL brought upon by orthodontic forces creates a local hypoxic condition [47]. Hypoxia-inducible gene transcription initiation factors, such

as HIF-1alpha, are stabilized on the pressure side of orthodontic tooth movement by the decrease in oxygen pressure. HIF-1alpha can subsequently enter into the nucleus of cells, in turn activating a cascade of pro-inflammatory molecules. One target gene of HIF-1 is cyclooxygenase (COX)-2 [48], the rate-limiting enzyme in the synthesis of prostaglandins (PGs) [49], including PGE_2, which is a potent nociceptor sensitizer among many. A variety of substances produced during the inflammation process can activate or sensitize nociceptors, the pain-sensing periphery nerve ending sensory organs, including tumor necrosis factor-α, IL-6, IL-1beta, bradykinin and ATP [44]. From there, painful signals are transmitted to the thalamus and subsequently are projected to the sensory cortex. During orthodontic tooth movement, we observe changes of gene expression patterns in the brain, such as the transcription

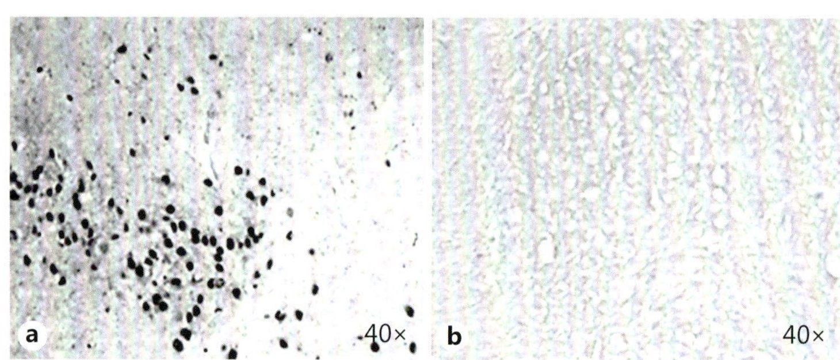

Fig. 4. SP is expressed in nerves located in the periodontal ligament. The neuropeptide SP is expressed by unmyelinated and thinly myelinated sensory nerve fibers. **a** Parasagittal histology section of a mouse maxilla stained by HE showing upper molars. **b** SP-expressing nerve fibers localized in the apical area of periodontal ligament (green) contrasted by nuclear Hoechst counterstain (blue).

Fig. 5. c-Fos induction in the trigeminal spinal nucleus. The immediate early gene c-Fos is associated with the processing of pain in the dorsal horns. **a** The expression of c-Fos is upregulated in the subnucleus caudalis (Vc) of the trigeminal spinal nucleus just minutes after the activation of peripheral sensory nerve fibers in an ipsilateral manner. **b** Contralateral side.

factor c-Fos, an apparent marker of pain processing by neurons regulating a variety of downstream genes [50]. Studies have found that orthodontic tooth movement induces c-Fos expression with a temporally and spatially distinct manner in the brain [51–56]. Tooth movement increases c-Fos expression in subnucleus caudalis (Vc) and dorsomedial part of subnucleus oralis (Vodm) of the spinal nucleus of trigeminal (fig. 5).

The pattern of c-Fos expression suggests the possible regions for modulation and transmission of nociceptive signals in the central nervous system. On the other hand, a recent study in rats [57] showed that orthodontic tooth movement significantly increases COX-2 expression in Vc with concomitant increased behavior associated with pain, while injection of a specific COX-2 inhibitor in the brain close to Vc of the brain stem significantly reduced behavior associated with pain in the animals. c-Fos is a positive regulator of COX-2 expression [58, 59]. In addition to neurons, inflammatory cells of the central nervous system are also activated in the Vc of the brain stem as a result of painful signals coming from the jaws, suggesting the development of local microenvironmental inflammation in the trigeminal spinal nucleus (fig. 6).

The nerves innervating the periodontium are not only 'signal wires' that transmit sensations, such as pain during orthodontic tooth movement, but also 'superhighways' that produce and transport inflammatory factors contributing to the remodeling of the periodontal ligament and alveolar bones throughout tooth movement.

Upon stimulation by inflammation mediators, such as bradykinin, hydrogen ions, prostaglandins and histamine, neuropeptides are released into surrounding tissues [60] in a process known as antidormic stimulation axon reflex. The neuropeptides, especially SP, act on the endothelial cells, mast cells and immune cells to enhance the inflammatory reaction, which is regarded as neurogenic inflammation [61]. SP and CGRP induce vasodilation and increase blood vessel

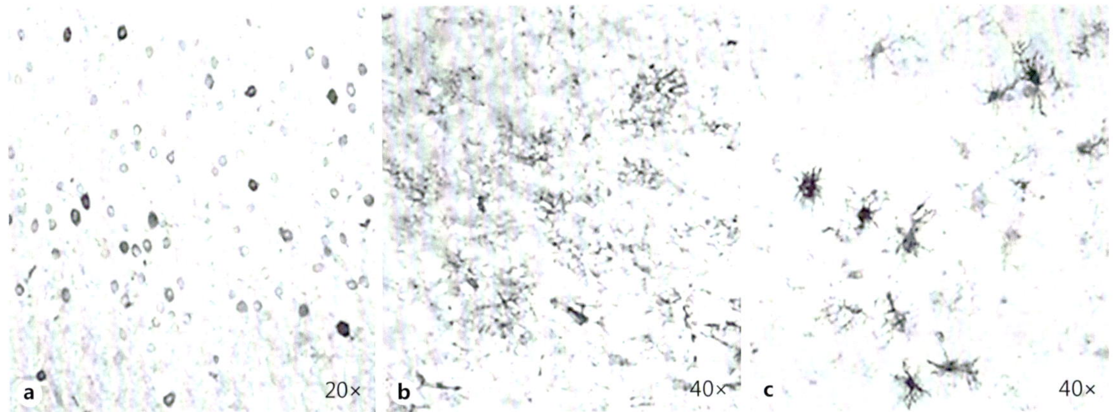

Fig. 6. Local inflammation in the trigeminal spinal nucleus as result of pain from the jaws. COX-2 expression in neurons of mice experiencing pain from the jaws (**a**), accompanied by activated astrocytes stained by the specific marker GFAP (**b**), and activated microglia stained by the specific marker MHC-II in the local microenvironment (**c**).

permeability when binding to their specific receptors on the endothelial cell surface [62, 63]. Mast cell degranulation is also induced by SP, causing further release of proinflammatory factors histamine and serotonin [64]. Some types of immune cells express receptors for neuropeptides and enable neuroimmune interactions. SP and CGRP are potent chemotactic agents for immune cells and are important for the recruitment of those cells [65, 66]. They also stimulate proliferation of lymphocytes [67, 68], promote production of immunoglobulins by B lymphocytes [69] and superoxide anion and prostaglandin production by macrophages [70–72]. The inflammation factors stimulated by neuropeptides will further trigger production and release of more neuropeptides. Therefore, a 'vicious cycle' of a noninfectious inflammatory reaction is formed by this mechanism. Neurogenic inflammation mediated by the neuropeptides not only intensifies, but also increases the field of the original inflammatory reaction and hyperalgesia. During orthodontic tooth movement, the expression of neuropeptides SP and CGRP are elevated in both periodontal tissues and the dental pulp, indicating the role of neurogenic pain in orthodontic treatment [33, 73–75].

The neuropeptides are important regulators in the cardiovascular system, respiratory system, gastrointestinal system and bones, etc. [61]. Afferent nerve endings containing SP and CGRP exist in the periosteum, PDL, dental pulp and temporomandibular joint as shown with immunohistochemistry staining [76–80]. Animal studies have shown that under orthodontic force, the expression of CGRP and SP are intensified, and the CGRP- and SP-positive fibers sprout to wider ranges in the PDL, dental pulp and marginal gingiva with a peak at 3 or 7 days after the application of orthodontic force, returning to normal after 7 days or remaining higher than normal 28 days after appliance removal [33, 37, 45, 75, 81, 82]. The discrepancies on the time course of neuropeptides' response to orthodontic force may be due to different types of appliances used in the studies [33]. Some CGRP-positive nerve fibers are in close proximity of bone resorptive lacunae during the active bone remodeling phase, suggesting the involvement of CGRP in bone remodeling [75]. The early intensification of CGRP and SP expression and sprouting of the nerve fibers containing these factors are concomitant with increased vascularity in the pulp and periodontal tissues [33]. On the other hand, denervation of dental tissues with inferior alveolar nerve sectioning causes reduced blood flow in the periodontal and pulp tissues [83], depleted tooth movement-induced elevation of CGRP expression and significantly reduced osteoclasts number and osteoclasts surface [84]. Together with the well-established proinflammatory functions of CGRP and SP, these studies strongly suggest that these neuropeptides play a crucial role in the inflammatory process and remodeling of PDL and bone during orthodontic treatment. Studies at the cellular and molecular levels demonstrate that CGRP receptors are expressed in both osteoblastic and osteoclastic lineage cells [85, 86]. In cell cultures, CGRP stimulates proliferation and differentiation of osteoblasts while inhibiting differentiation and function of osteoclasts [85–89]. SP also has osteogenic effects [90, 91], but seems to stimulate osteoclast function and bone resorption [92]. More studies should focus on the regulation of bone metabolism by neuropeptides and other neurogenic factors in order to understand the role of the neural tissues in orthodontic tooth movement which may lead to clinically applicable methods to manage pain associated with orthodontic treatment and to control the rate of tooth movement.

Pain Management

Management of pain and discomfort during orthodontic treatment includes pharmacological and nonpharmacological methods. Pharmacological intervention remains the most common option, and the most widely used method is nonsteroidal anti-inflammatory drugs (NSAIDs), including acetylsalicylic acid (Aspirin), ibuprofen (Advil, Motrin), flurbiprofen (Ansaid), naproxen sodium (Aleve, Anaprox, Anaprox DS, Naprelan, Naprosyn) and tenoxicam (Tilcotil). Acetaminophen (Tylenol) is also commonly employed. The NSAIDs reduce pain by inhibiting COX-1 and COX-2 and reducing PG production [49]. The mechanism of the analgesic action of acetaminophen is not completely clear, but recent studies showed that it selectively inhibits COX-2 [93], and its metabolites target transient receptor potential cation channel, subfamily A, member 1 in the spinal cord to inhibit signal transduction from the dorsal horn [94]. One meta-analysis showed that ibuprofen significantly reduced pain at 6 and 24 h after initial archwire placement compared with placebo, while aspirin and acetaminophen were similarly effective in pain relief compared with ibuprofen [95]. Another meta-analysis largely agreed with the results except that ibuprofen showed a statistically significant pain-relieving effect compared with placebo at 2 and 6 h, but not at 24 h, after separators and archwire placement [96]. Other NSAIDs were also shown to be effective to relieve orthodontic pain, including Valdecoxib [97] and Tenoxicam [98]. It was proposed that ibuprofen should be taken both preoperatively and postoperatively to effectively reduce pain [96]. PGs are important molecules in causing pain induced by inflammation. On the other hand, PGs, especially PGE_1 and PGE_2, are factors crucial for remodeling of the alveolar bone, which is indispensable for orthodontic tooth movement. In both animal and human studies, local administration of PGE_1 or PGE_2 significantly accelerated orthodontic tooth movement [99, 100]. Therefore, though NSAIDs are effective pain relievers during orthodontic treatment, they have been shown to delay tooth movement [101–103], which may be due to inhibition of bone remodeling rate. It was also shown that the NSAID indomethacin significantly exacerbated IL-1beta-induced matrix metalloproteinases (MMPs) production by endothelial cells. MMPs are enzymes responsible for degradation of collagen. Increased level of MMPs may cause aberrant remodeling of periodontal structures and affect normal orthodontic tooth movement [104].

Nonpharmacological interventions are also effective in relieving pain during orthodontic treatment. Transcutaneous electrical nerve stimulation was shown to reduce pain at 24, 36 and 48 h after initial archwire placement compared with placebo treatment or control [105]. Thera-bite (add company name and location) wafer chewing alleviated pain in slightly more than half of orthodontic patients, while the rest reported increased discomfort. The opposing effects of thera-bite wafer chewing seemed to be related to the amount of time used daily with longer time chewing resulting in pain relief while less time resulting in more pain, or the reduction of pain was due to placebo effect [106]. Lim et al. [107] found that irradiating the buccal side of the roots of teeth receiving separators with low level laser for 30 or 60 s could lower the level of pain on the second and the third day, although the effect was not statistically significant. Vibratory stimulation significantly reduced pain level from 2 h to 3 days after archwire placement compared with the control group if used before the unset of pain. If used after the onset of pain, however, pain would be exacerbated by vibration [108]. Bartlett et al. [109] found that with a structured telephone call from a health-care provider, which conveyed care and reassurance or just expressed attention, there was a significant reduction in self-reported pain in patients who had initial archwire placement. Cognitive behavioral therapy, which was consisted with guided imaginary, activity pacing, relaxation training, assistance in dealing with pain-related anxiety and problem solving, was as effective as ibuprofen in pain relieving for orthodontic patients after initial insertion of archwire [110]. It is possible that the pain alleviating effects of a structured telephone call and cognitive behavioral therapy is due to reduction of patients' anxiety and subjective perception of pain.

References

1 Kvam E, Gjerdet NR, Bondevik O: Traumatic ulcers and pain during orthodontic treatment. Community Dent Oral Epidemiol 1987;15:104–107.
2 Lew KK: Attitudes and perceptions of adults towards orthodontic treatment in an Asian community. Community Dent Oral Epidemiol 1993;21:31–35.
3 Scheurer PA, Firestone AR, Burgin WB: Perception of pain as a result of orthodontic treatment with fixed appliances. Eur J Orthod 1996;18:349–357.
4 O'Connor PJ: Patients' perceptions before, during, and after orthodontic treatment. J Clin Orthod 2000;34:591–592.
5 Brown DF, Moerenhout RG: The pain experience and psychological adjustment to orthodontic treatment of preadolescents, adolescents, and adults. Am J Orthod Dentofacial Orthop 1991;100:349–356.
6 Jones M, Chan C: The pain and discomfort experienced during orthodontic treatment: a randomized controlled clinical trial of two initial aligning arch wires. Am J Orthod Dentofacial Orthop 1992;102:373–381.
7 Ngan P, Kess B, Wilson S: Perception of discomfort by patients undergoing orthodontic treatment. Am J Orthod Dentofacial Orthop 1989;96:47–53.
8 Bondemark L, Fredriksson K, Ilros S: Separation effect and perception of pain and discomfort from two types of orthodontic separators. World J Orthod 2004;5:172–176.
9 Erdinc AM, Dincer B: Perception of pain during orthodontic treatment with fixed appliances. Eur J Orthod 2004;26:79–85.
10 Fernandes LM, Ogaard B, Skoglund L: Pain and discomfort experienced after placement of a conventional or a superelastic NiTi aligning archwire. A randomized clinical trial. J Orofac Orthop 1998;59:331–339.
11 Haynes S: Discontinuation of orthodontic treatment relative to patient age. J Dent 1974;2:138–142.
12 Oliver RG, Knapman YM: Attitudes to orthodontic treatment. Br J Orthod 1985;12:179–188.
13 Jones ML, Richmond S: Initial tooth movement: force application and pain – a relationship? Am J Orthod 1985;88:111–116.
14 Ogura M, et al: Pain intensity during the first 7 days following the application of light and heavy continuous forces. Eur J Orthod 2009;31:314–319.
15 Luppanapornlarp S, et al: Interleukin-1beta levels, pain intensity, and tooth movement using two different magnitudes of continuous orthodontic force. Eur J Orthod 2010;32:596–601.
16 Stewart FN, Kerr WJ, Taylor PJ: Appliance wear: the patient's point of view. Eur J Orthod 1997;19:377–382.
17 Sergl HG, Klages U, Zentner A: Pain and discomfort during orthodontic treatment: causative factors and effects on compliance. Am J Orthod Dentofacial Orthop 1998;114:684–691.
18 Cioffi I, et al: Pain perception following first orthodontic archwire placement – thermoelastic vs. superelastic alloys: a randomized controlled trial. Quintessence Int 2012;43:61–69.
19 Scott P, et al: Perception of discomfort during initial orthodontic tooth alignment using a self-ligating or conventional bracket system: a randomized clinical trial. Eur J Orthod 2008;30:227–232.

20 Fleming PS, et al: Pain experience during initial alignment with a self-ligating and a conventional fixed orthodontic appliance system. A randomized controlled clinical trial. Angle Orthod 2009; 79:46–50.

21 Tecco S, et al: Prevalence and type of pain during conventional and self-ligating orthodontic treatment. Eur J Orthod 2009;31:380–384.

22 Wu AK, et al: A comparison of pain experienced by patients treated with labial and lingual orthodontic appliances. Eur J Orthod 2010;32:403–407.

23 Needleman HL, et al: Reports of pain by children undergoing rapid palatal expansion. Pediatr Dent 2000;22:221–226.

24 Cureton SL: Headgear and pain. J Clin Orthod 1994;28:525–530.

25 Pancherz H and Anehus-Pancherz M: The effect of continuous bite jumping with the Herbst appliance on the masticatory system: a functional analysis of treated class II malocclusions. Eur J Orthod 1982;4:37–44.

26 Deguchi T, et al: Clinical evaluation of temporomandibular joint disorders (TMD) in patients treated with chin cup. Angle Orthod 1998;68:91–94.

27 Jones ML: An investigation into the initial discomfort caused by placement of an archwire. Eur J Orthod 1984;6:48–54.

28 Rahim-Williams B, et al: A quantitative review of ethnic group differences in experimental pain response: do biology, psychology, and culture matter? Pain Med 2012;13:522–540.

29 Bergius M, Kiliaridis S, Berggren U: Pain in orthodontics. A review and discussion of the literature. J Orofac Orthop 2000;61:125–137.

30 Krishnan V: Orthodontic pain: from causes to management – a review. Eur J Orthod 2007;29:170–179.

31 Chapman CR, Turner JA: Psychological control of acute pain in medical settings. J Pain Symptom Manage 1986;1:9–20.

32 Litt MD: A model of pain and anxiety associated with acute stressors: distress in dental procedures. Behav Res Ther 1996;34:459–476.

33 Vandevska-Radunovic V, Kvinnsland S, Kvinnsland IH: Effect of experimental tooth movement on nerve fibres immunoreactive to calcitonin gene-related peptide, protein gene product 9.5, and blood vessel density and distribution in rats. Eur J Orthod 1997;19:517–529.

34 Kvinnsland I, Heyeraas KJ, Byers MR: Effects of dental trauma on pulpal and periodontal nerve morphology. Proc Finn Dent Soc 1992;88(suppl 1):125–132.

35 Wakisaka S, et al: Immunoelectron microscopic study on neuropeptide Y in the periodontal ligament of the incisor following peripheral nerve injury to the inferior alveolar nerve in the rat. Brain Res 1996;729:259–263.

36 Nishikawa S: Systemic labeling and visualization of dental sensory nerves by the novel fluorescent marker AM1–43. Anat Sci Int 2006;81:181–186.

37 Norevall LI, Matsson L, Forsgren S: Main sensory neuropeptides, but not VIP and NPY, are involved in bone remodeling during orthodontic tooth movement in the rat. Ann N Y Acad Sci 1998;865:353–359.

38 Sasano T, et al: Direct evidence of parasympathetic vasodilatation in cat periodontal ligament. J Periodontal Res 1996;31:556–562.

39 Barde YA: The nerve growth factor family. Prog Growth Factor Res 1990;2:237–248.

40 Thoenen H, Barde YA, Edgar D: The role of nerve growth factor (NGF) and related factors for the survival of peripheral neurons. Adv Biochem Psychopharmacol 1981;28:263–273.

41 McMahon SB: NGF as a mediator of inflammatory pain. Philos Trans R Soc Lond B Biol Sci 1996;351:431–440.

42 Smeyne RJ, et al: Severe sensory and sympathetic neuropathies in mice carrying a disrupted Trk/NGF receptor gene. Nature 1994;368:246–249.

43 Priestley JV, et al: Regulation of nociceptive neurons by nerve growth factor and glial cell line derived neurotrophic factor. Can J Physiol Pharmacol 2002;80:495–505.

44 Coutaux A, et al: Hyperalgesia and allodynia: peripheral mechanisms. Joint Bone Spine 2005;72:359–371.

45 O'Hara AH, et al: Immunohistochemical detection of nerve growth factor and its receptors in the rat periodontal ligament during tooth movement. Arch Oral Biol 2009;54:871–878.

46 Ye XD, Laties AM, Stone RA: Peptidergic innervation of the retinal vasculature and optic nerve head. Invest Ophthalmol Vis Sci 1990;31:1731–1737.

47 Park HJ, et al: Hypoxia inducible factor-1alpha directly induces the expression of receptor activator of nuclear factor-kappaB ligand in periodontal ligament fibroblasts. Mol Cells 2011;31:573–578.

48 Lee JJ, et al: Hypoxia activates the cyclooxygenase-2-prostaglandin E synthase axis. Carcinogenesis 2010;31:427–434.

49 Vane JR: Inhibition of prostaglandin synthesis as a mechanism of action for aspirin-like drugs. Nat New Biol 1971;231:232–235.

50 Harris JA: Using c-fos as a neural marker of pain. Brain Res Bull 1998;45:1–8.

51 Kato J, et al: Induction of Fos protein in the rat trigeminal nucleus complex during an experimental tooth movement. Arch Oral Biol 1994;39:723–726.

52 Yamashiro T, et al: c-fos expression in the trigeminal sensory complex and pontine parabrachial areas following experimental tooth movement. Neuroreport 1997;8:2351–2353.

53 Fujiyoshi Y, et al: The difference in temporal distribution of c-Fos immunoreactive neurons between the medullary dorsal horn and the trigeminal subnucleus oralis in the rat following experimental tooth movement. Neurosci Lett 2000;283:205–208.

54 Watanabe M, et al: Expression of c-Fos protein in the trigeminal nuclear complex resulting from quantified force application to the rat molar. J Oral Rehabil 2003;30:1128–1137.

55 Magdalena CM, et al: C-fos expression in rat brain nuclei following incisor tooth movement. J Dent Res 2004;83:50–54.

56 Novaes AP, da Rocha MJ, Leite-Panissi CR: Tooth movement activates the central amygdala and the lateral hypothalamus by the magnitude of the force applied. Angle Orthod 2010;80:111–115.

57 Gao Y, Duan YZ: Increased COX2 in the trigeminal nucleus caudalis is involved in orofacial pain induced by experimental tooth movement. Anat Rec (Hoboken) 2010;293:485–491.

58 Huang H, et al: Parathyroid hormone induction of cyclooxygenase-2 in murine osteoblasts: role of the calcium-calcineurin-NFAT pathway. J Bone Miner Res 2010;25:819–829.

59 Seo JH, Kim H, Kim KH: Cyclooxygenase-2 expression by transcription factors in Helicobacter pylori-infected gastric epithelial cells: comparison between HP 99 and NCTC 11637. Ann N Y Acad Sci 2002;973:477–480.

60 Richardson JD, Vasko MR: Cellular mechanisms of neurogenic inflammation. J Pharmacol Exp Ther 2002;302:839–845.

61 Maggi CA: Tachykinins and calcitonin gene-related peptide (CGRP) as co-transmitters released from peripheral endings of sensory nerves. Prog Neurobiol 1995;45:1–98.

62 Maggi CA, et al: Peripheral effects of neurokinins: functional evidence for the existence of multiple receptors. J Auton Pharmacol 1987;7:11–32.

63 Gray DW, Marshall I: Human alpha-calcitonin gene-related peptide stimulates adenylate cyclase and guanylate cyclase and relaxes rat thoracic aorta by releasing nitric oxide. Br J Pharmacol 1992;107:691–696.

64 Assem ES, et al: Substance P and Arg-Pro-Lys-Pro-NH-C12-H25-induced mediator release from different mast cell subtypes of rat and guinea-pig. Immunopharmacology 1989;17:119–128.

65 Marasco WA, Showell HJ, Becker EL: Substance P binds to the formylpeptide chemotaxis receptor on the rabbit neutrophil. Biochem Biophys Res Commun 1981;99:1065–1072.

66 Foster CA, et al: Calcitonin gene-related peptide is chemotactic for human T lymphocytes. Ann N Y Acad Sci 1992;657:397–404.

67 Casini A, et al: Effects of calcitonin gene-related peptide (CGRP), neurokinin A and neurokinin A (4–10) on the mitogenic response of human peripheral blood mononuclear cells. Naunyn Schmiedebergs Arch Pharmacol 1989;339:354–358.

68 Payan DG, Brewster DR, Goetzl EJ: Specific stimulation of human T lymphocytes by substance P. J Immunol 1983;131:1613–1615.

69 Bost KL, Pascual DW: Substance P: a late-acting B lymphocyte differentiation cofactor. Am J Physiol 1992;262:C537–C545.

70 Brunelleschi S, et al: Tachykinins activate guinea-pig alveolar macrophages: involvement of NK2 and NK1 receptors. Br J Pharmacol 1990;100:417–420.

71 Brunelleschi S, et al: Evidence for tachykinin NK-2B-like receptors in guinea-pig alveolar macrophages. Life Sci 1992;51:PL177–PL181.

72 Brunelleschi S, et al: Enhanced responsiveness of ovalbumin-sensitized guinea-pig alveolar macrophages to tachykinins. Br J Pharmacol 1992;107:964–969.

73 Yamaguchi M, Yoshii M, Kasai K: Relationship between substance P and interleukin-1beta in gingival crevicular fluid during orthodontic tooth movement in adults. Eur J Orthod 2006;28:241–246.

74 Giannopoulou C, Dudic A, Kiliaridis S: Pain discomfort and crevicular fluid changes induced by orthodontic elastic separators in children. J Pain 2006;7:367–376.

75 Saito I, et al: Responses of calcitonin gene-related peptide-immunopositive nerve fibres in the periodontal ligament of rat molars to experimental tooth movement. Arch Oral Biol 1991;36:689–692.

76 Hill EL, Elde R: Calcitonin gene-related peptide-immunoreactive nerve fibers in mandibular periosteum of rat: evidence for primary afferent origin. Neurosci Lett 1988;85:172–178.

77 Kato J, et al: The distribution of vasoactive intestinal polypeptides and calcitonin gene-related peptide in the periodontal ligament of mouse molar teeth. Arch Oral Biol 1990;35:63–66.

78 Hill EL, Elde R: Distribution of CGRP-, VIP-, D beta H-, SP-, and NPY-immunoreactive nerves in the periosteum of the rat. Cell Tissue Res 1991;264:469–480.

79 Kido MA, et al: Distribution of substance P and calcitonin gene-related peptide-like immunoreactive nerve fibers in the rat temporomandibular joint. J Dent Res 1993;72:592–598.

80 Jacobsen EB, Fristad I, Heyeraas KJ: Nerve fibers immunoreactive to calcitonin gene-related peptide, substance P, neuropeptide Y, and dopamine beta-hydroxylase in innervated and denervated oral tissues in ferrets. Acta Odontol Scand 1998;56:220–228.

81 Kvinnsland I, Kvinnsland S: Changes in CGRP-immunoreactive nerve fibres during experimental tooth movement in rats. Eur J Orthod 1990;12:320–329.

82 Norevall LI, Forsgren S, Matsson L: Expression of neuropeptides (CGRP, substance P) during and after orthodontic tooth movement in the rat. Eur J Orthod 1995;17:311–325.

83 Vandevska-Radunovic V, Kvinnsland IH, Kvinnsland S: Effect of inferior alveolar nerve axotomy on periodontal and pulpal blood flow subsequent to experimental tooth movement in rats. Acta Odontol Scand 1998;56:57–64.

84 Yamashiro T, et al: Inferior alveolar nerve transection inhibits increase in osteoclast appearance during experimental tooth movement. Bone 2000;26:663–669.

85 Granholm S, Lundberg P, Lerner UH: Expression of the calcitonin receptor, calcitonin receptor-like receptor, and receptor activity modifying proteins during osteoclast differentiation. J Cell Biochem 2008;104:920–933.

86 Wang L, et al: Calcitonin-gene-related peptide stimulates stromal cell osteogenic differentiation and inhibits RANKL induced NF-kappaB activation, osteoclastogenesis and bone resorption. Bone 2010;46:1369–1379.

87 Granholm S, Henning P, Lerner UH: Comparisons between the effects of calcitonin receptor-stimulating peptide and intermedin and other peptides in the calcitonin family on bone resorption and osteoclastogenesis. J Cell Biochem 2011;112:3300–3312.

88 Wang YS, et al: Osteogenic potential of human calcitonin gene-related peptide alpha gene-modified bone marrow mesenchymal stem cells. Chin Med J (Engl) 2011;124:3976–3981.

89 Akopian A, et al: Effects of CGRP on human osteoclast-like cell formation: a possible connection with the bone loss in neurological disorders? Peptides 2000;21:559–564.

90 Shih C, Bernard GW: Neurogenic substance P stimulates osteogenesis in vitro. Peptides 1997;18:323–326.

91 Kook YA, et al: Effects of substance P on osteoblastic differentiation and heme oxygenase-1 in human periodontal ligament cells. Cell Biol Int 2009;33:424–428.

92 Mori T, et al: Substance P regulates the function of rabbit cultured osteoclast; increase of intracellular free calcium concentration and enhancement of bone resorption. Biochem Biophys Res Commun 1999;262:418–422.

93 Hinz B, Cheremina O, Brune K: Acetaminophen (paracetamol) is a selective cyclooxygenase-2 inhibitor in man. FASEB J 2008;22:383–390.

94 Andersson DA, et al: TRPA1 mediates spinal antinociception induced by acetaminophen and the cannabinoid delta(9)-tetrahydrocannabiorcol. Nat Commun 2011;2:551.

95 Xiaoting L, Yin T, Yangxi C: Interventions for pain during fixed orthodontic appliance therapy. A systematic review. Angle Orthod 2010;80:925–932.

96 Angelopoulou MV, Vlachou V, Halazonetis DJ: Pharmacological management of pain during orthodontic treatment: a meta-analysis. Orthod Craniofac Res 2012;15:71–83.

97 Young AN, et al: Evaluation of pre-emptive valdecoxib therapy on initial archwire placement discomfort in adults. Angle Orthod 2006;76:251–259.

98 Arantes GM, et al: Tenoxicam controls pain without altering orthodontic movement of maxillary canines. Orthod Craniofac Res 2009;12:14–19.

99 Yamasaki K, Shibata Y, Fukuhara T: The effect of prostaglandins on experimental tooth movement in monkeys (*Macaca fuscata*). J Dent Res 1982;61:1444–1446.

100 Yamasaki K, et al: Clinical application of prostaglandin E1 (PGE1) upon orthodontic tooth movement. Am J Orthod 1984;85:508–518.

101 Arias OR, Marquez-Orozco MC: Aspirin, acetaminophen, and ibuprofen: their effects on orthodontic tooth movement. Am J Orthod Dentofacial Orthop 2006;130:364–370.

102 Kehoe MJ, et al: The effect of acetaminophen, ibuprofen, and misoprostol on prostaglandin E_2 synthesis and the degree and rate of orthodontic tooth movement. Angle Orthod 1996;66:339–349.

103 Chumbley AB, Tuncay OC: The effect of indomethacin (an aspirin-like drug) on the rate of orthodontic tooth movement. Am J Orthod 1986;89:312–314.

104 Kyrkanides S, O'Banion MK, Subtelny JD: Nonsteroidal anti-inflammatory drugs in orthodontic tooth movement: metalloproteinase activity and collagen synthesis by endothelial cells. Am J Orthod Dentofacial Orthop 2000;118:203–209.

105 Roth PM, Thrash WJ: Effect of transcutaneous electrical nerve stimulation for controlling pain associated with orthodontic tooth movement. Am J Orthod Dentofacial Orthop 1986;90:132–138.

106 Hwang JY, et al: Effectiveness of therabite wafers in reducing pain. J Clin Orthod 1994;28:291–292.

107 Lim HM, Lew KK, Tay DK: A clinical investigation of the efficacy of low level laser therapy in reducing orthodontic postadjustment pain. Am J Orthod Dentofacial Orthop 1995;108:614–622.

108 Marie SS, Powers M, Sheridan JJ: Vibratory stimulation as a method of reducing pain after orthodontic appliance adjustment. J Clin Orthod 2003;37:205–208; quiz 203–204.

109 Bartlett BW, et al: The influence of a structured telephone call on orthodontic pain and anxiety. Am J Orthod Dentofacial Orthop 2005;128:435–441.

110 Wang J, et al: Cognitive behavioral therapy for orthodontic pain control: a randomized trial. J Dent Res 2012;91:580–585.

Dr. Stephanos Kyrkanides
Department of Orthodontics and Pediatric Dentistry, Stony Brook University
Rockland Hall Rm 114
Stony Brook, NY 11794-8701 (USA)
E-Mail Kyrkanides@gmail.com

Kantarci A, Will L, Yen S (eds): Tooth Movement. Front Oral Biol. Basel, Karger, 2016, vol 18, pp 75–79
DOI: 10.1159/000351901

Osteoclastogenesis and Osteogenesis during Tooth Movement

S. Susan Baloul

The Forsyth Institute, Cambridge, Mass., USA

Abstract

It is a well-known concept that bone remodeling occurs during orthodontic tooth movement. The orthodontic literature is vastly full of information about the changes occurring on the periodontal ligament level. However, changes occurring in the alveolar bone are being elucidated. The purpose of this chapter is to present some of the studies describing the bone changes associated with orthodontic tooth movement. Initiation of osteoclastogenesis requires inflammation in the adjacent area. Tissue biomarker RANKL responds to the compressive forces. Conversely, an increase in osteoprotegrin biomarker causes a decrease in RANKL and inhibits tooth movement. Osteocyte activity during tooth movement is not well understood. Emerging studies are showing the effect of osteocytes on orthodontic tooth movement. Nitric oxide (NO), produced by osteocytes, is an important regulator of bone response to loading and has been shown to mediate osteoclast activity. iNOS (which produces NO) has been shown to mediate inflammation-induced bone resorption on the compression side. Several molecules have been linked to osteogenesis in tooth movement: TGF-β, BSP, BMPs and epidermal growth factor. Osteogenesis on the tension side is not well understood. Studies have shown increase in the expression of Runx2 on the tension side. Additionally, eNOS (produces NO) mediates bone formation on the tension side. The concept of osteoclastogenesis and osteogenesis is being unraveled.

© 2016 S. Karger AG, Basel

Alveolar Bone Response during Tooth Movement

During tooth movement, two bone activities occur adjacent to the tooth that is undergoing the orthodontic migration: resorption and deposition. Alveolar bone resorption occurs on the side toward which the tooth is moving during the physiologic tooth movements. Simultaneously, reconstruction of the ligamentous support between tooth and bone takes place. Histologically, active bone resorption is observed by the presence of osteoclasts residing in scattered resorptive lacunae on the alveolar bone wall [1]. The osteoclasts are recruited from adjacent marrow space [2]. Tooth movement is hindered until the osteoclasts remove the necrotic tissue. This phenomenon is observed clinically as a lag (delay) period as described by Graber and Vanarsdall [3]. This was similarly demonstrated in a rat model [4] where the tooth movement experi-

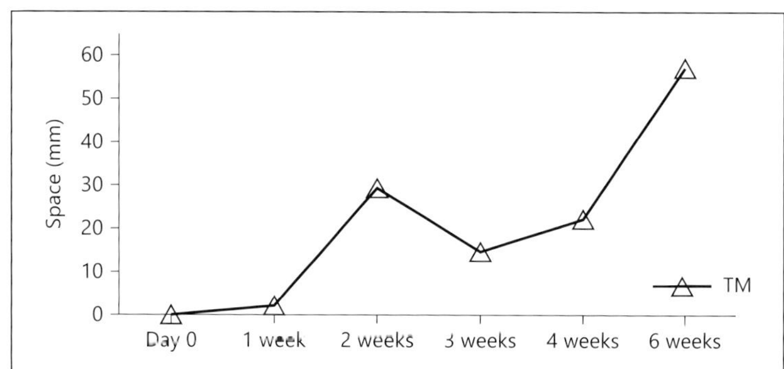

Fig. 1. Space changes during orthodontic tooth movement.

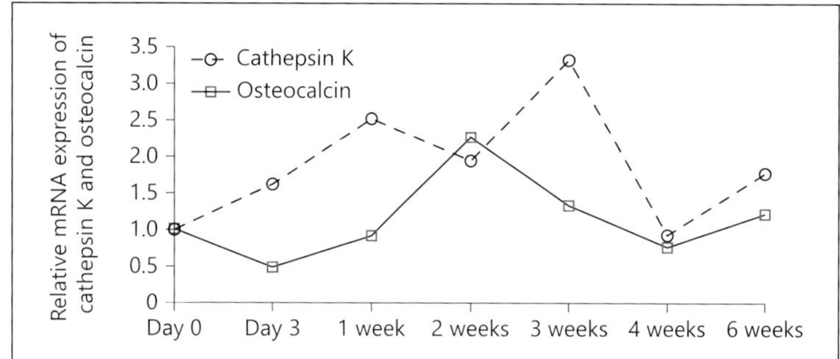

Fig. 2. Osteoclastic biomarker (cathepsin K) and osteoblastic biomarker (osteocalcin) pathways during orthodontic tooth movement in a rat model.

enced a lag of between two and four weeks after initiation of orthodontic force as shown in figure 1. During this period, bone resorption is high, as seen by the upregulation in the osteoclastic bone marker cathepsin K, while bone apposition is low as shown by the downregulation of the osteoblastic bone marker osteocalcin (fig. 2). Once the bone resorption ceases, the cells housed in Howship's lacunae deposit new bone layers where periodontal fibrils become embedded. Histological studies demonstrated the reestablishment of the fiber attachment mechanism on the alveolar bone wall [5], root cementum [6–10], and secondary dentin [11] in the resorption sites.

Alveolar bone deposition occurs on the side opposite the direction in which the tooth is moving. The tissue reaction to this movement is by bone apposition and periodontal fiber rearrangement [1]. New Sharpey's fibers are formed and incorporated into the existing fibers [12]. The timing of the events occurring at the compression sites in orthodontic tooth movement [5] is consistent with the bone remodeling cycle described by Frost [13]. Microcracks at the compression sites, caused by fatigue or trauma, are important in initiating orthodontic bone remodeling [14, 15]. The capability of displacement from the crack tearing osteocyte cell processes may lead to secretion of bioactive molecules into the extracellular matrix and may therefore cause a response [16]. During extensive bone remodeling in orthodontics, bone formation tends to be slower than bone resorption. This possibly could explain the clinical findings such as tooth mobility and radiographic widening in the periodontal ligament (PDL) space observed in orthodontic tooth movement, and signify that remodeling is the prevalent turnover process at orthodontic compression sites [17].

Osteoclastogenesis in Orthodontic Tooth Movement

Application of force during orthodontic tooth movement leads to the initiation of osteoclastogenesis. Two associated changes occur during osteoclastogenesis. First, tissue damage occurs with further production of inflammatory processes in the PDL. Second, alveolar process deformation takes place. A few days after force application, the first osteoclast progenitor cells appear at the compression sites in the alveolar crest vasculature and marrow spaces, and the PDL space widens [2, 18]. Osteoclasts appear in higher quantity at the compression sites compared to tension sites [19]. In addition, proinflammatory cytokines such as IL-6, IL-8 and TNF-α are produced, which suggests the importance of inflammation in initiating osteoclastogenesis during tooth movement [20, 21].

Changes also occur in the tooth-supporting tissue biomarkers RANK, RANKL and osteoprotegrin during tooth movement [22]. RANKL stimulates and inhibits osteoprotegrin during tooth movement [23]. RANKL is upregulated in response to compressive forces [24] through a prostaglandin endogenous 2 (PGE_2) pathway supporting the role of osteoclastogenesis. RANKL-mediated osteoclastogenesis and tooth movement are both inhibited by local osteoprotegrin gene transfer [25]. It has been shown that an increase in RANKL and a decrease in osteoprotegrin has a negative impact on tooth movement therapy in terms of causing severe root resorption [26].

During the period of 5–7 days following force activation [27], osteoclasts are cleared from compression sites. This may be due to osteoclast apoptosis followed by secondary necrosis [28]. A second pathway for osteoclast death occurs through integrins (specific receptor-like molecules), focal adhesion proteins and cytoskeleton (activation of MAPK, p38, and JNK/SAPK protein kinase pathways), by force activation. This pathway causes osteoclast apoptosis by amplifying the signal and activating caspases. The type of force stimulus and cell phenotype determines whether the osteoclast undergoes apoptosis followed by secondary necrosis or just apoptosis [29].

The role of osteocytes, the predominant bone cell in alveolar bone during orthodontic movement, has not been well studied in the orthodontic literature. Osteocytes are well-equipped to facilitate bone adaptation to loading [30]. The physiological changes in periodontal tissue during orthodontic tooth movement affect the activity, metabolism, and communication of osteocytes [31]. Nitric oxide (NO) is an important regulator of bone response to mechanical loading. It is produced by endothelial nitric oxide synthase (eNOS) or inducible nitric oxide synthase (iNOS) [32], and has been shown to: mediate adaptive bone formation [33] and osteoclast activity [34], and prevents osteocyte apoptosis [35, 36]. Several authors have shown that inhibition of NO production increases osteoclastogenesis [37, 38]. Orthodontic force results in strain within the bone giving rise to fluid flow leading to production of NO by osteocytes [39]. Additionally, it has been suggested that iNOS mediates inflammation-induced bone resorption in the compression area [39]. It has been shown that osteocytes and osteoclasts undergo apoptosis at orthodontic compression sites [31]. However, this concept is not fully understood.

Osteogenesis in Orthodontic Tooth Movement

The type of orthodontic force determines the osteoblast recruitment and tensile strains determine the osteogenic activity. Static loads have no role in skeletal osteogenesis and that short periods (bouts) of loading above certain threshold steer osteogenesis [40]. Strain rates, amplitude and duration of these loads are important in osteogenesis [40]. It is believed that physical activities including mastication, speech and swallowing make the orthodontic loads as bouts type of loading. Without these physical loading changes, one would look at orthodontic loading as static [17]. It has been shown that tensile strains stimulate the proliferation of the osteoblast progenitor cells in the PDL. This leads to bone formation and inhibition of bone resorption. Molecules linked to osteogenesis in orthodontic tooth movement are: TGF-β [41], BSP [42], BMPs [43] and epidermal growth factor [44].

The mechanism of osteogenesis during orthodontic tooth movement on the tension side is not well understood. Once orthodontic force is applied, the mechanical forces are first received by the fibroblasts in the PDL. An in vitro study has shown that cyclic strain results in an increased osteogenic gene expression in PDL fibroblasts [45]. The expression of Runx2 and the phosphorylation of extracellular signal-regulated kinases 1/2 (pERK1/2) have been shown to increase on the tension side in an orthodontic tooth movement model [46]. The concept of regulation of bone remodeling during orthodontic movement on the tension side was first described by Diercke et al. [47], who demonstrated the role of ephrin-B2-EphB4 signaling between PDLF and osteoblasts at the tension sites of bone remodeling during orthodontic movement. Additionally, eNOS which produces NO (described previously) has been shown to mediate bone formation in the tension area during orthodontic tooth movement [39].

Osteoclastogenesis and osteogenesis associated with tooth movement are two separate concepts orchestrated simultaneously facilitating orthodontic tooth movement. More studies need to be done for understanding the concept of alveolar bone remodeling during orthodontic tooth movement.

References

1 Moyers RE: Handbook of Orthodontics. Chicago, Year Book Medical Publishers, 1988.

2 Rody WJ Jr, King GJ, Gu G: Osteoclast recruitment to sites of compression in orthodontic tooth movement. Am J Orthod Dentofac Orthoped 2001;120:477–489.

3 Graber TM, Vanarsdall RL: Orthodontics: current principles and techniques. St Louis, Mosby, 2000.

4 Baloul SS, Gerstenfeld LC, Morgan EF, Carvalho RS, Van Dyke TE, Kantarci A: Mechanism of action and morphologic changes in the alveolar bone in response to selective alveolar decortication-facilitated tooth movement. Am J Orthod Dentofac Orthop 2011;139(4 suppl):S83–S101.

5 King GJ, Keeling SD, McCoy EA, Ward TH: Measuring dental drift and orthodontic tooth movement in response to various initial forces in adult rats. Am J Orthod Dentofac Orthoped 1991;99:456–465.

6 Rygh P: Ultrastructural changes of the periodontal fibers and their attachment in rat molar periodontium incident to orthodontic tooth movement. Scand J Dent Res 1973;81:467–480.

7 Rygh P: Elimination of hyalinized periodontal tissues associated with orthodontic tooth movement. Scand J Dent Res 1974;82:57–73.

8 Rygh P: Hyalinization of the periodontal ligament incident to orthodontic tooth movement. Den Norske Tannlaegeforenings Tidende 1974;84:352–357.

9 Brudvik P, Rygh P: The repair of orthodontic root resorption: an ultrastructural study. Eur J Orthod 1995;17:189–198.

10 Casa MA, Faltin RM, Faltin K, Arana-Chavez VE: Root resorption on torqued human premolars shown by tartrate-resistant acid phosphatase histochemistry and transmission electron microscopy. Angle Orthodontist 2006;76: 1015–1021.

11 Nixon CE, Saviano JA, King GJ, Keeling SD: Histomorphometric study of dental pulp during orthodontic tooth movement. J Endod 1993;19:13–16.

12 Garant PR, Cho MI: Autoradiographic evidence of the coordination of the genesis of Sharpey's fibers with new bone formation in the periodontium of the mouse. J Periodontal Res 1979;14:107–114.

13 Frost HM: The biology of fracture healing: an overview for clinicians. Part I. Clin Orthop 1989;248:283–293.

14 Verna C, Dalstra M, Lee TC, Cattaneo PM, Melsen B: Microcracks in the alveolar bone following orthodontic tooth movement: a morphological and morphometric study. Eur J Orthod 2004;26: 459–467.

15 Galley SA, Michalek DJ, Donahue SW: A fatigue microcrack alters fluid velocities in a computational model of interstitial fluid flow in cortical bone. J Biomech 2006;39:2026–2033.

16 Hazenberg JG, Freeley M, Foran E, Lee TC, Taylor D: Microdamage: a cell transducing mechanism based on ruptured osteocyte processes. J Biomech 2006;39:2096–2103.

17 Wise GE, King GJ: Mechanisms of tooth eruption and orthodontic tooth movement. J Dent Res 2008;87:414–434.

18 Yokoya K, Sasaki T, Shibasaki Y: Distributional changes of osteoclasts and preosteoclastic cells in periodontal tissues during experimental tooth movement as revealed by quantitative immunohistochemistry of H(+)-ATPase. J Dent Res 1997;76:580–587.

19 Kawarizadeh A, Bourauel C, Zhang D, Gotz W, Jager A: Correlation of stress and strain profiles and the distribution of osteoclastic cells induced by orthodontic loading in rat. Eur J Oral Sci 2004;112:140–147.

20 Alhashimi N, Frithiof L, Brudvik P, Bakhiet M: Orthodontic tooth movement and de novo synthesis of proinflammatory cytokines. Am J Orthod Dentofac Orthoped 2001;119:307–312.

21 Lee B: Force and tooth movement. Aust Orthod J 2007;23:155.

22 Oshiro T, Shiotani A, Shibasaki Y, Sasaki T: Osteoclast induction in periodontal tissue during experimental movement of incisors in osteoprotegerin-deficient mice. Anat Rec 2002;266:218–225.

23 Kanzaki H, Chiba M, Takahashi I, Haruyama N, Nishimura M, Mitani H: Local OPG gene transfer to periodontal tissue inhibits orthodontic tooth movement. J Dent Res 2004;83:920–925.

24 Kanzaki H, Chiba M, Shimizu Y, Mitani H: Periodontal ligament cells under mechanical stress induce osteoclastogenesis by receptor activator of nuclear factor kappaB ligand up-regulation via prostaglandin E_2 synthesis. J Bone Miner Res 2002;17:210–220.

25 Kanzaki H, Chiba M, Sato A, Miyagawa A, Arai K, Nukatsuka S, Mitani H: Cyclical tensile force on periodontal ligament cells inhibits osteoclastogenesis through OPG induction. J Dent Res 2006;85:457–462.

26 Yamaguchi M, Aihara N, Kojima T, Kasai K: RANKL increase in compressed periodontal ligament cells from root resorption. J Dent Res 2006;85:751–756.

27 King GJ, Keeling SD, Wronski TJ: Histomorphometric study of alveolar bone turnover in orthodontic tooth movement. Bone 1991;12:401–409.

28 Noxon SJ, King GJ, Gu G, Huang G: Osteoclast clearance from periodontal tissues during orthodontic tooth movement. Am J Orthod Dentofac Orthoped 2001;120:466–476.

29 Hsieh MH, Nguyen HT: Molecular mechanism of apoptosis induced by mechanical forces. Int Rev Cytol 2005;245:45–90.

30 Cowin SC, Moss-Salentijn L, Moss ML: Candidates for the mechanosensory system in bone. J Biomech Eng 1991;113:191–197.

31 Hamaya M, Mizoguchi I, Sakakura Y, Yajima T, Abiko Y: Cell death of osteocytes occurs in rat alveolar bone during experimental tooth movement. Calcif Tissue Int 2002;70:117–126.

32 van't Hof RJ, Ralston SH: Nitric oxide and bone. Immunology 2001;103:255–261.

33 Fox SW, Chambers TJ, Chow JW: Nitric oxide is an early mediator of the increase in bone formation by mechanical stimulation. Am J Physiol 1996;270:E955–E960.

34 van't Hof RJ, Armour KJ, Smith LM, Armour KE, Wei XQ, Liew FY, Ralston SH: Requirement of the inducible nitric oxide synthase pathway for IL-1-induced osteoclastic bone resorption. Proc Natl Acad Sci U S A 2000;97:7993–7998.

35 Tan SD, Kuijpers-Jagtman AM, Semeins CM, Bronckers AL, Maltha JC, Von den Hoff JW, Everts V, Klein-Nulend J: Fluid shear stress inhibits TNF-alpha-induced osteocyte apoptosis. J Dent Res 2006;85:905–909.

36 Tan SD, Bakker AD, Semeins CM, Kuijpers-Jagtman AM, Klein-Nulend J: Inhibition of osteocyte apoptosis by fluid flow is mediated by nitric oxide. Biochem Biophys Res Commun 2008;369:1150–1154.

37 Collin-Osdoby P, Rothe L, Bekker S, Anderson F, Osdoby P: Decreased nitric oxide levels stimulate osteoclastogenesis and bone resorption both in vitro and in vivo on the chick chorioallantoic membrane in association with neoangiogenesis. J Bone Miner Res 2000;15:474–488.

38 Tan SD, de Vries TJ, Kuijpers-Jagtman AM, Semeins CM, Everts V, Klein-Nulend J: Osteocytes subjected to fluid flow inhibit osteoclast formation and bone resorption. Bone 2007;41:745–751.

39 Tan SD, Xie R, Klein-Nulend J, van Rheden RE, Bronckers AL, Kuijpers-Jagtman AM, Von den Hoff JW, Maltha JC: Orthodontic force stimulates eNOS and iNOS in rat osteocytes. J Dent Res 2009;88:255–260.

40 Forwood MR, Turner CH: Skeletal adaptations to mechanical usage: results from tibial loading studies in rats. Bone 1995;17(4 suppl):197S–205S.

41 Brady TA, Piesco NP, Buckley MJ, Langkamp HH, Bowen LL, Agarwal S: Autoregulation of periodontal ligament cell phenotype and functions by transforming growth factor-beta1. J Dent Res 1998;77:1779–1790.

42 Domon S, Shimokawa H, Yamaguchi S, Soma K: Temporal and spatial mRNA expression of bone sialoprotein and type I collagen during rodent tooth movement. Eur J Orthod 2001;23:339–348.

43 Mitsui N, Suzuki N, Maeno M, Yanagisawa M, Koyama Y, Otsuka K, Shimizu N: Optimal compressive force induces bone formation via increasing bone morphogenetic proteins production and decreasing their antagonists production by Saos-2 cells. Life Sci 2006;78:2697–2706.

44 Guajardo G, Okamoto Y, Gogen H, Shanfeld JL, Dobeck J, Herring AH, Davidovitch Z: Immunohistochemical localization of epidermal growth factor in cat paradental tissues during tooth movement. Am J Orthod Dentofac Orthoped 2000;118:210–219.

45 Wescott DC, Pinkerton MN, Gaffey BJ, Beggs KT, Milne TJ, Meikle MC: Osteogenic gene expression by human periodontal ligament cells under cyclic tension. J Dent Res 2007;86:1212–1216.

46 Kawarizadeh A, Bourauel C, Gotz W, Jager A: Early responses of periodontal ligament cells to mechanical stimulus in vivo. J Dent Res 2005;84:902–906.

47 Diercke K, Kohl A, Lux CJ, Erber R: Strain-dependent up-regulation of ephrin-B2 protein in periodontal ligament fibroblasts contributes to osteogenesis during tooth movement. J Biol Chem 2011;286:37651–37664.

S. Susan Baloul
Private Practice
55 Main Street
Framington, MA 01702 (USA)
E-Mail Susan.Baloul@gmail.com

Kantarci A, Will L, Yen S (eds): Tooth Movement. Front Oral Biol. Basel, Karger, 2016, vol 18, pp 80–91
DOI: 10.1159/000382048

Nonsurgical Methods for the Acceleration of the Orthodontic Tooth Movement

Konstantinia Almpani · Alpdogan Kantarci

Forsyth Institute, Cambridge, Mass., USA

Abstract

While acceleration of the orthodontic tooth movement by surgical techniques has been shown to be effective for decades, noninvasive and nonsurgical methods have always been preferred by both the clinicians and the patients. These techniques have ranged from application of biological molecules to innovative technologies such as resonance vibration, cyclic forces, light electrical currents, magnetic field forces, low-intensity laser irradiation and low-level light therapy. Endogenously produced biologicals have been tested based on their roles in the turnover of alveolar bone in response to orthodontic tooth movement as well as during wound healing. The premise behind this approach is that these exogenously applied compounds will mimic their counterparts produced in vivo. Meanwhile, technologies tested so far target these pathways for the acceleration of the orthodontic tooth movement. All these approaches have shown favorable outcomes with varying success. This chapter presents the current knowledge and a discussion over their limitations with an emphasis on the mechanism of action for each technique.   © 2016 S. Karger AG, Basel

One of the main advantages of comprehensive orthodontic treatment is being a noninvasive dental procedure. Thus, any additional surgical procedures for orthodontic purposes are generally undesirable, by both patients and orthodontists. For that reason, nonsurgical techniques for the acceleration of tooth movement have been extensively explored. As recent research has demonstrated, there is a multifactorial sequence of events occurring during the tooth movement process. The synthesis, release as well as the role of various inflammatory mediators, neurotransmitters, growth factors and other cytokines in response to applied mechanical forces have been elucidated. Many of these endogenous factors have also been involved in orthodontic treatment movement acceleration research, and the effect of their local and/or systemic administration has been tested, mainly in animal models, with variable results.

In addition, physical stimulation techniques, which have been previously reported to enhance and accelerate tissue regeneration in other medical fields, have also become increasingly popular in orthodontic movement acceleration research. Specifically, the effect of resonance vibration, cyclic forces, light electrical currents, magnetic field forces, low-intensity (low-level) laser irradiation therapy (LILT) and low-level light therapy (LLLT) application on the orthodontic tooth movement rate have been examined in various studies.

Systemic/Local Administration of Chemical Substances

Epidermal Growth Factor
It has long been demonstrated that epidermal growth factor (EGF) has catabolic effects on bone. In an organ culture study, high concentrations of EGF stimulated bone resorption in fetal rat long bone [1, 2]. Administration of EGF at high doses to rats caused an elevation of osteoclastic cell density on the trabecular bone surface [3]. Consistently, in transgenic mice overexpressing human EGF, thinner bones were observed [4], suggesting an imbalance in bone modeling or remodeling. In fact, exogenous EGF administration had an additive effect on the rate of osteoclast recruitment producing faster bone resorption and tooth movement [5]. Recently, it has been shown that EGF plays a role in mediating the ability of human bone marrow stromal cells to induce osteoclast differentiation [6, 7]. Moreover, the regulatory role of EGF in fibrous tissue remodeling in the periodontal ligament (PDL) has also been demonstrated [8].

Regarding the influence of EGF administration on the orthodontic tooth movement rate, studies in animals have shown that EGF administration has an additive effect on the rate of osteoclast genesis and recruitment, which leads to faster bone resorption and orthodontic movement acceleration [5, 9]. Moreover, EGF has also been identified as a participant in the bone-remodeling process during orthodontic movement [10–12].

The complex role of EGF in orthodontic tooth movement remains to be explored even further. The formation of more efficient and safe administration animal models is essential before the conduction of any trials in humans.

Parathyroid Hormone
Parathyroid hormone (PTH) is the major hormone regulating bone remodeling and calcium homeostasis. By increasing the concentration of calcium in the blood, it stimulates bone resorption [13–17]. Although continuous elevation of PTH leads to bone loss, intermittent short elevations of the hormone level can be anabolic for bone [18]. Experimental and clinical data has shown that daily administrations of PTH led to increases in bone mass, mineral density and strength [19].

The effect of PTH on orthodontic tooth movement has been studied in rats [20–22]. A significant stimulation of the rate of orthodontic tooth movement by exogenous PTH administration appeared to occur in a dose-dependent manner. However, this effect was only visible when the hormone was more or less continuously applied, either by systemic infusion [20] or frequent local delivery [21, 22].

It is well known that chronic elevation of PTH leads to pathological changes in multiple organs, especially the kidneys and bones [20, 23]. The short-term studies that have been conducted until the present have not been able to determine the long-term effects of PTH at the dose used to accelerate tooth movement, especially regarding the kidney function and bone condition. Thus, safety remains a serious concern for its clinical application in orthodontic treatment [24]. Nevertheless, local injections of PTH in slow-release formulations did not significantly affect the rate of tooth movement in animals [22]. Consequently, the safety and efficiency of this systemic factor in orthodontic movement acceleration remain to be further investigated.

1,25-Dihydroxyvitamin D_3
Another agent that has been identified as an important factor in orthodontic tooth movement is 1,25-dihydroxycholeciferol (1,25-DHCC) [25, 26]. This agent is a biologically active form of vitamin D and has a potent role in calcium homeostasis. A decrease in the serum calcium level stimulates secretion of PTH, which in turn increases the excretion of PO_4^{-3}, reabsorption of Ca^{2+} from the kidneys, and hydroxylation of 25-hydroxycholecaliferol to 1,25-DHCC. The latter molecule

has been shown to be a potent stimulator of bone resorption by inducing differentiation of osteoclasts from their precursors. It is also implicated in increasing the activity of existing osteoclasts. In addition to bone-resorbing activity, 1,25-DHCC is known to stimulate bone mineralization and osteoblastic cell differentiation in a dose-dependent manner.

Animal studies have demonstrated that local injections of 1,25-DHCC accelerate orthodontic tooth movement by about 1.2- to 2.5-fold [25–27]. Histological examinations also showed that 1,25-DHCC stimulates the formation of osteoclasts in a dose-dependent manner [26] and causes significantly more alveolar bone resorption [25]. No obvious clinical, microscopic or biochemical side effects have been noted until now, but the safe use of this systemic factor in orthodontic movement should be further investigated. Nevertheless, the current way of administration of 1,25-DHCC with the use of frequent injections is also decreasing the clinical practicality of this factor in orthodontic patients.

L-Thyroxine

Thyroid hormones play an imperative role in the regulation of cellular metabolism, proliferation and differentiation [28]. L-Thyroxine is a synthetic thyroid hormone that is chemically identical to thyroxine, which is naturally secreted by the thyroid gland and has been used to treat thyroid hormone deficiency and occasionally to prevent the recurrence of thyroid cancer. Furthermore, thyroxine affects intestinal calcium absorption and, therefore, is indirectly involved in bone turnover. Hyperthyroidism or thyroxine medication can lead to osteoporosis [29].

Because of the ability of thyroid hormones to act on the metabolism of nearly every cell in the body and especially of their indirect involvement in bone turnover [30–32], the possible effect of 80-thyroxine on orthodontic tooth movement has also been examined [33] in a relevant study on rats. The results showed that administration of 20 µg/kg i.p./day L-thyroxine significantly increased the amount of orthodontic tooth movement. The extent of root resorption as seen from scanning electron micrographs appeared to decrease with thyroxine administration. Verna et al. [34] examined whether the rate of orthodontic tooth movement is influenced by the general bone turnover capacity in another rat model. They obtained a high turnover by the general administration of L-thyroxine. The rate of tooth movement was higher in cases of high bone turnover and smaller in the rats with low bone turnover, in comparison to normal animals. This finding is consistent with a generally more rapid tooth movement found in animals with high turnover caused by secondary hyperparathyroidism [35–37]. Because of the fact that thyroxine medication can lead to osteoporosis, the seriousness of safety issues regarding its use for orthodontic purposes is quite high. Its use is still on an experimental level in animal models, and no human trials have been conducted so far.

Osteocalcin

Osteocalcin (OC) is the most abundant noncollagenous matrix protein in bone [38]. Because of its strong capacity to associate with Ca^{2+} and hydroxyapatite, OC is a negative regulator for mineral apposition and bone formation [39–42]. In addition, OC is proposed to be a chemoattractant for progenitor/mature osteoclasts [43–45].

In studies in rats, it was demonstrated that local injections of purified rat OC accelerated the rate and increased the total amount of tooth movement [38, 46]. Histological examination revealed that this acceleration of tooth movement was caused by an enhanced recruitment of osteoclasts. No other side effects were reported, and no apparent macroscopic inflammation could be detected at the injection sites. Due to the restricted amount of existing data, no further conclusions can be currently formed regarding the effect of OC on the rate of tooth movement.

Prostaglandins

Prostaglandins (PGs) are an interesting group of multifunctional regulators during orthodontic tooth movement. These lipids are synthesized by arachidonic acid by the sequential actions of cyclooxygenase (COX) and respective synthases. PGs are released in response to various stimuli and have multiple physiological effects, two of which include the amplification of the effects of cytokines and bone metabolism, largely due to COX-2 induction. PGs have the ability to recruit inflammatory cells and enhance the expression of inflammation-related genes. Furthermore, they can either facilitate or suppress tissue remodeling and regulate bone metabolism, stimulating both bone resorption and deposition [24, 47]. Among the PGs that had been found to affect bone metabolism (E_1, E_2, A_1 and $F_{2\alpha}$), PGE_2 is the one that stimulates osteoblastic cell differentiation and new bone formation, coupling bone resorption in vitro [48].

The clinical effect of exogenous PGs on orthodontic tooth movement has been an object of research for a lot of years. Several animal studies have concluded on the fact that local application of PGE_1, PGE_2, analogs of PGE_1, PGE_2 or thromboxane A_2 can increase the speed of orthodontic tooth movement [27, 49–53].

Local submucosal injections of PGE_1 in patients were also successful in accelerating orthodontic tooth movement by 1.6-fold [54]. Respectively, orthodontic tooth movement is impaired by nonsteroidal anti-inflammatory drugs, the compounds that inhibit the COX-1 and COX-2 enzymes that catalyze the rate-limiting step of PG formation [55, 56].

The main side effect associated with local injection of PGs is hyperalgesia, due to the release of noxious agents such as histamine, bradykinin, serotonin, acetylcholine and substance P, from nerve endings both peripherally and centrally [57, 58]. This indicates that although PGs enhance the tooth movement process, their side effects are still too serious to consider its clinical use in orthodontic patients. Recent research trends are directed towards combining local anesthetics with PGs, in order to reduce pain while injected locally, but research in this regard is still in its preliminary phase. Moreover, another concern that has been repeatedly reported by different researchers is an increased risk of root resorption that seems to be concomitant with their administration [57]. Consequently, further research is required regarding their use in orthodontic treatment.

Gene Transfer Therapy

With the aid of gene therapy, it is possible to deliver a gene to a given group of target cells, which allows the inserted gene product to be locally expressed constitutively. In this way, higher and more constant levels of protein expression can be produced in a certain area. Local tooth movement-accelerating factors can be 'administered' with this technique. The advantages in this case are that the local concentration of the active factor remains effective due to its continuous production by the treated cells and that systemic side effects are avoided at the same time [59, 60].

The role of cytokines of the receptor activator of nuclear factor κ ligand (RANKL)-RANK/osteoprotegerin (OPG) system in inducing bone remodeling has already been demonstrated [61]. The tumor necrosis factor-related ligand RANKL and its two receptors RANK and OPG have been shown to be involved in this remodeling process. RANKL is a downstream regulator of osteoclast formation and activation, through which many hormones and cytokines produce their osseoresorptive effect. In the bone system, RANKL is expressed on the osteoblast cell lineage and exerts its effect by binding the RANK receptor on osteoclast lineage cells. This binding leads to rapid differentiation of hematopoietic osteoclast precursors to mature osteoclasts. OPG is a decoy receptor produced by osteoblastic cells, which compete with RANK for RANKL binding. The biological effects of OPG on bone cells include inhibition of terminal stages of osteoclast differentiation, suppression of activation of matrix osteoclasts and induction of apoptosis. Thus, bone remodeling is controlled by a balance between RANK-RANKL binding and OPG production.

Oshiro et al. [62] reported that RANKL induction was also observed in the periodontal tissue of the orthodontically moving tooth, and the RANK-RANKL regulation system was confirmed even in the site-specific bone remodeling that occurred during the orthodontic tooth movement.

A previous study in rats demonstrated that transfer of the RANKL gene to a periodontal tissue activated osteoclastogenesis and accelerated orthodontic tooth movement without producing any systemic effects [63]. Iglesias-Linares et al. [64] also demonstrated in a more recent study that RANKL gene transfer was a more efficient technique for the reduction of total treatment duration in comparison to alveolar corticotomy.

In conclusion, gene transfer is a new, promising therapeutic modality that is currently under rapid development. It offers an alternative method to deliver proteins to a given target tissue, which, in turn, can enhance osteoclast recruitment and lead to accelerated orthodontic treatment movement. The results from its applications until now are very encouraging. Nonetheless, further research is required for the identification of all the biological factors involved and in order to be in a position to fully control the outcome of this kind of therapy. This is a prerequisite step for the determination of the safety and efficacy of gene therapy in live organisms.

Relaxin

Relaxin is a naturally occurring hormone with the primary function of widening the pubic symphysis during childbirth and has been proven to be present in craniofacial structures, such as calvarial sutures [65]. Furthermore, relaxin influences many other physiological processes such as collagen turnover, angiogenesis and antifibrosis in both males and females [66]. The latter actions suggested that relaxin might influence orthodontic tooth movement through alterations of the PDL [66].

In a study in rats, Liu et al. [67] examined the effect of a local administration of human relaxin in orthodontic tooth movement. According to their results, relaxin had a positive influence on the orthodontic movement rate. Nevertheless, in another rat model study, Madan et al. [66] reported that relaxin does not affect either the rate or the amount of tooth movement. Regardless, they observed that it can reduce the level of PDL organization, reduce PDL mechanical strength and increase tooth mobility at early time points.

McGorray et al. [68] reported, in a randomized, blinded clinical trial in human subjects comparing a group who received relaxin injections weekly for 8 weeks with those who received placebo injections, that the pattern and amount of tooth movement did not differ. However, they also stated that the local doses of relaxin might have been too low to affect tooth movement. Based on these results, it is more likely that relaxin would find its most significant clinical application in reducing the tendency for post-orthodontic tooth relapse and not in the enhancement of orthodontic tooth movement.

Resonance Vibration

Resonance vibration is based on a frequency equal to the natural frequency of an object, causing the largest amplitude of vibration of this object [24]. The initial response of cells to mechanical stress in vitro appears within 30 min [69, 70]. In a recent study, Nishimura et al. [71] attempted to activate these initial responses at the cellular level by applying resonance vibrational stimulation to a tooth and its periodontal tissue. They applied resonance vibration (60 Hz) to the first molars in rats for 8 min, once a week during orthodontic movement. According to their results, resonance vibration increased tooth movement by 15% compared with the controls, stimulating more expression of RANKL and osteoclast formation in the PDL. Due to the natural frequency of the vibration applied, there is no collateral damage to the periodontal tissues or root resorption of the treated teeth.

Ultrasonic vibration is also a form of vibrational stimulation that is similar to resonance vibration. It has been reported that ultrasonic vibration accelerates tooth movement too [72]. However, ultrasonic vibration of teeth might be associated with certain hazards, such as thermal damage to the dental pulp [73].

Recently, a novel cyclical force device, 'AcceleDent', has been marketed, with claims that it may increase the rate of orthodontic movement. However, it provides vibration with only one fixed frequency (4 Hz), and there is still no peer-reviewed or long- term study on the biological or the clinical effects of the appliance [74].

Electrical Currents

Another tool that has been used in order to accelerate orthodontic tooth movement is electricity. Since the early observation of Fukada and Yasuda [75] that electric potentials are generated by the application of force to bone, many investigators used external electricity to enhance osteogenesis [76]. It was demonstrated that when electrodes are placed into bone osteogenesis will occur around the negative electrode when the current level is between 5 and 20 μA, while resorption of bone may occur around the positive electrode (anode) [76].

Davidovitch et al. [77] reported in an animal study that electric stimulation may accelerate bone turnover and, therefore, orthodontic tooth movement. Based on the results of another animal study, Hashimoto [78] concluded that micropulsed electrical stimulation might play a role in the efficient remodeling of alveolar bone and in the efficient remodeling of alveolar bone and in

inducing more rapid tooth movement. Specifically, he observed changes in the periodontal tissue, accelerated tooth movement, wider areas of bone deposition and larger amounts of newly formed bone, increasing over time in amount, on the tension side, a larger number of osteoblasts on the tension side and more tartrate-resistant acid phosphatase-positive mononuclear and multinuclear cells on the compression side.

In a clinical study with orthodontic patients, Kim et al. [79] also demonstrated that an electrical current (20 μA for 5 h daily) was capable of accelerating orthodontic tooth movement. Currently, the existing level of evidence is not enough to support whether electrical current could be effective in accelerating orthodontic tooth movement with safety in humans [80, 81].

Static or Pulsed Magnetic Field

Magnetic fields, including static magnetic field [82, 83] and pulsed electromagnetic field [82, 84, 85], have been proven to increase the speed of orthodontic tooth movement in animal studies. Histological analyses have suggested that alveolar bone remodeling is activated under the influence of magnetic fields as activities of bone cells are elevated, and new bone deposition is increased on the tension side [82, 84, 85]. Hyalinization in the PDL was also reduced in the group treated with the static magnetic field, which also contributed to accelerated tooth movement [83].

According to a more recent study in orthodontic patients, exposure of canines to a pulsed electromagnetic field (1 Hz), during their retraction to first premolar extraction sites, had as a result the acceleration of their movement [86].

However, there were also studies that not only did not agree with the above results in terms of tooth movement rate, but also reported increased root resorption of the treated teeth, prompting concerns about the effectiveness and safety of this method [87]. Therefore, further studies are required to determine the effect of magnetic fields on tooth movement. In addition, the source of electricity still poses a problem for the clinical use of this method, too. Microfabricated biocatalytic fuel cells (enzyme batteries) might resolve this issue in the future [88].

Low-Intensity Laser Irradiation Therapy

Various biostimulatory effects of LILT have been shown, including effects on wound healing [89], fibroblastic [90] and chondral [91] proliferation, collagen synthesis [92] and nerve regeneration [93]. In particular, the acceleration of bone regeneration by laser treatment has been the focus of many studies [94]. In the field of orthodontics, low-energy laser irradiation has been utilized for several types of orthodontic applications, such as the reduction of postappliance adjustment pain [95] or the treatment of traumatic ulcers in the oral mucosa [96].

Aluminum-gallium-arsenide (Ga-Al-As) diode lasers are the ones that are currently most used for these interventions and have been proven to have a higher depth of tissue penetration in comparison to other modalities, therefore providing the clinicians with a suitable penetrative instrument with great efficiency [97]. The exact mechanism of laser-cell interaction is still to be investigated. The stimulation of photoreceptors in the mitochondrial respiratory chain, changes in cellular ATP levels and cell membrane stabilization have been discussed [98]. It is generally accepted that laser effects on cells are wavelength and dose dependent. The existence of a 'window of specificity' at certain wavelengths and energy dosages has been postulated. Therefore, different wavelengths and energy outputs of these laser devices have been tested in different studies.

Saito and Shimizu [99] observed that LILT with a Ga-Al-As infrared diode laser device (wavelength: 830 nm; continuous wave at 100 mW; power density: 35.3 J/s/cm^2) can accelerate bone regeneration in the midpalatal suture of rats during rapid palatal expansion and stimulate the synthesis of collagen, which is the major matrix protein in bone.

Kawasaki and Shimizu [23] also reported that orthodontic movement of low-intensity laser-irradiated rat teeth was 30% faster than that of the teeth in a control nonirradiated group of rats. They also used a Ga-Al-As infrared diode laser device (wavelength: 830 nm; output power: 100–700 mW, variable; total energy corresponding to a 9-min exposure: 54.0 J). Enhanced bone formation was observed on the pressure side and an increased number of osteoclasts on the compression side, logically as a result of cellular stimulation promoted by low-energy laser irradiation. These results agree with the reports of numerous other animal studies on the stimulation capacity of LILT regarding the alveolar bone remodeling and subsequent acceleration of the velocity of orthodontic tooth movement [100–103].

In another study with rats, Fujita et al. [104] examined the effect of LILT and light-emitting diode (LED) irradiation on orthodontic tooth movement. According to their results, the amount and rate of tooth movement were significantly greater in the laser irradiation group (day 3: 2.2-fold; day 4: 2.0-fold; day 7: 1.5-fold) compared with the nonirradiation and LED irradiation groups.

According to the results of the relative histological analyses, most studies have reported that LILT stimulates alveolar bone remodeling activities as indicated by the increased numbers and functions of osteoclasts and osteoblasts [23, 100, 102, 103, 105] as well as by molecular markers such as matrix metalloproteinase-9, cathepsin K, $\alpha_v\beta_3$-integrin [106], the RANK/RANKL/OPG system [104, 105, 107, 108] and basic fibroblast growth factor [109].

On the other hand, Limpanichkul et al. [110] reported that LILT with the use of Ga-Al-As (wavelength: 860 nm; continuous wave power output: 100 mW; power density: 1.11 W/cm^2; energy dose: 2.3 J/point; energy density: 25 J/cm^2/site) was too low to express either a stimulatory effect or inhibitory effect on the rate of orthodontic tooth movement. Similar results have also been reported by a few other clinical studies like the one from Gama et al. [111] (wavelength: 790 nm; energy dose: 4.5 J/cm^2). The discrepancies may be explained by the different treatment protocols used in these studies, including the wavelengths of the lasers, irradiation doses, locations and frequencies [24].

Altan et al. [105] aimed to evaluate the effects of the 820-nm diode laser (output power: 100 mW) in orthodontic movement in rats, comparing different energy doses at the same time (3.18 W/cm^2, 1,717.2 J/cm^2 vs. 3.18 W/cm^2, 477 J/cm^2). The number of osteoclasts, osteoblasts, inflammatory cells, capillary vascularization and new bone formation were found to be significantly increased in the first group (3.18 W/cm^2, 1,717.2 J/cm^2). Immunohistochemical staining findings also showed that RANKL immunoreactivity was stronger in the same group. Based on these findings they also concluded that LILT accelerates the bone-remodeling process during orthodontic tooth movement.

Cruz et al. [112] were the first to publish research results on the effect of LILT on the duration of dental movement in humans. They conducted a split-mouth design study with 11 subjects, between 12 and 18 years of age, who received mechanical activation for the retraction of their upper canine teeth in the space of extracted premolars every 30 days. Each tooth was receiving the same mechanical activation, but one of them was also receiving LILT with a diode laser emitting light at 780 nm, during 10 s at 20 mW, 5 J/cm^2, on 4 days of each month. According to their results, orthodontic movement of the treated teeth was accelerated due to the use of laser radiation. Since then, more clinical studies in humans have also revealed a significantly positive effect of low-intensity laser radiation on the acceleration of orthodontic tooth movement, like the ones from Youssef et al. [113] (wavelength: 809 nm; output power: 100 mW), Sousa et al. [114] (wavelength: 780 nm; output power: 20 mW;

power density: 5 J/cm^2) and Genc et al. [115] (wavelength: 808 nm; output power: 20 mW; power density: 0.71 J/cm^2).

In conclusion, the biostimulant effects of LILT have been indicated in many studies. In the case of clinical studies in humans, the subjects were mainly adolescents and young adults, between 12 and 23 years of age. No studies in older adults have been published. However, more research is still necessary in order to establish the most efficient protocol that would enhance the effect and reduce the frequency of irradiation sessions, in order to make this treatment more clinically applicable.

Photobiomodulation or Low-Level Light Therapy

Photobiomodulation is an emerging medical and dental technique in which exposure to light or LEDs stimulates cellular function leading to beneficial clinical effects. This technique is known as low-level light therapy or LLLT. The light spectrum may vary, but it falls in the infrared range. A Ga-Al-As diode laser produces coherent light, whereas the light produced by the LED is incoherent. This technique has been based on the fact that cytochrome oxidase c or complex IV – an enzyme which mediates the synthesis of ATP in cells – is upregulated by infrared light [116]. During tooth movement, higher ATP availability boosts cell metabolism, leading to an increased remodeling process and accelerated tooth movement [117, 118]. LLLT may also be enhancing orthodontic tooth movement due to increased vascular activity, which is also promoted by light [119] and contributes to a more rapid bone turnover [120].

Previous studies have shown that the impact of the LLLT is also dependent on the wavelength and intensity of the emitted light [121]. Until now, there has been a number of studies suggesting an enhanced impact of LLLT in the acceleration of orthodontic tooth movement [116, 122, 123]. The results of a large multicenter clinical trial in 90 orthodontic patients, aged from 10 to 36 years of age [118], however, demonstrated that when photobiomodulation was applied (wavelength: 850 nm; power density: 60 mW/cm^2 for 20/day or 30/day or 60 min/week; total energy densities: 72, 108 and 216 J/cm^2), the rate of tooth movement significantly increased during the initial alignment phase. In particular, the rates of tooth movement in the alignment phase were 1.12 mm/week for those in the photobiomodulation treatment group compared to 0.49 mm in the control group.

Nevertheless, according to the results of Fujita et al. [104], infrared LED irradiation (wavelength: 850 nm; output power: 75 mW; total energy dose: 54.0 J/cm^2) did not stimulate the velocity of tooth movement or osteoclastogenesis in rats. Vinck et al. [120] also reported – in an in vitro study – that infrared LED irradiation did not stimulate the proliferation of fibroblasts obtained from chicken embryos.

Conclusively, larger and longer clinical trials are required in order to be able to assess the validity of LLLT, the long-term stability of the produced outcomes and any potential adverse effects. Moreover, more research studies on a mo-lecular level are also needed that would lead to a deeper understanding of the biological mechanisms involved, which would simplify and optimize the clinical applications of LLLT.

Conclusions

Nonsurgical techniques are more preferable for orthodontic patients, since any kind of surgery, no matter how minor; is not free from side effects and usually comes with an additional cost. However, the local administration of systemic regulatory factors for that purpose has been linked with an increased risk for root resorption and pain. Further investigations are required to determine the correct dosage, frequency of administration and, especially, the possible local and systemic side effects of their use.

Physical stimulation techniques, though, appear to be less prone to adverse effects. They are noninvasive, pain free and in general more attractive to orthodontic patients and clinicians. Nevertheless, more efficient application protocols and scientific evidence are necessary before their introduction to the clinical practice.

References

1 Raisz LG, et al: Direct stimulation of bone resorption by epidermal growth factor. Endocrinology 1980;107:270–273.

2 Lorenzo JA, et al: Effects of DNA and prostaglandin synthesis inhibitors on the stimulation of bone resorption by epidermal growth factor in fetal rat long-bone cultures. J Clin Invest 1986;77:1897–1902.

3 Marie PJ, Hott M, Perheentupa J: Effects of epidermal growth factor on bone formation and resorption in vivo. Am J Physiol 1990;258:E275–E281.

4 Chan SY, Wong RW: Expression of epidermal growth factor in transgenic mice causes growth retardation. J Biol Chem 2000;275:38693–38698.

5 Saddi KR, et al: Epidermal growth factor in liposomes may enhance osteoclast recruitment during tooth movement in rats. Angle Orthod 2008;78:604–609.

6 Normanno N, et al: Gefitinib inhibits the ability of human bone marrow stromal cells to induce osteoclast differentiation: implications for the pathogenesis and treatment of bone metastasis. Endocr Relat Cancer 2005;12:471–482.

7 Normanno N, Gullick WJ: Epidermal growth factor receptor tyrosine kinase inhibitors and bone metastases: different mechanisms of action for a novel therapeutic application? Endocr Relat Cancer 2006;13:3–6.

8 Kimura H, et al: EGF positively regulates the proliferation and migration, and negatively regulates the myofibroblast differentiation of periodontal ligament-derived endothelial progenitor cells through MEK/ERK- and JNK-dependent signals. Cell Physiol Biochem 2013;32:899–914.

9 Alves JB, et al: Local delivery of EGF-liposome mediated bone modeling in orthodontic tooth movement by increasing RANKL expression. Life Sci 2009;85:693–699.

10 Dolce C, et al: Effects of sialoadenectomy and exogenous EGF on molar drift and orthodontic tooth movement in rats. Am J Physiol 1994;266:E731–E738.

11 Cao QL, et al: Comparison of long bone repair in tibia by vascularized fibular grafting of different sides (in Chinese). Zhongguo Xiu Fu Chong Jian Wai Ke Za Zhi 2002;16:109–111.

12 Gao Q, et al: Expression of epidermal growth factor and epidermal growth factor receptor in rat periodontal tissues during orthodontic tooth movement. Zhonghua Kou Qiang Yi Xue Za Zhi 2002;37:294–296.

13 Takahashi N, et al: Osteoclast-like cell formation and its regulation by osteotropic hormones in mouse bone marrow cultures. Endocrinology 1988;122:1373–1382.

14 Perry HM 3rd, et al: Partial characterization of a parathyroid hormone-stimulated resorption factor(s) from osteoblast-like cells. Endocrinology 1989;125:2075–2082.

15 Collin P, Guenther HL, Fleisch H: Constitutive expression of osteoclast-stimulating activity by normal clonal osteoblast-like cells: effects of parathyroid hormone and 1,25-dihydroxyvitamin D_3. Endocrinology 1992;131:1181–1187.

16 Weir EC, et al: Macrophage colony-stimulating factor release and receptor expression in bone cells. J Bone Miner Res 1993;8:1507–1518.

17 McSheehy PM, Chambers TJ: Osteoblast-like cells in the presence of parathyroid hormone release soluble factor that stimulates osteoclastic bone resorption. Endocrinology 1986;119:1654–1659.

18 Potts JT, Gardella TJ: Progress, paradox, and potential: parathyroid hormone research over five decades. Ann N Y Acad Sci 2007;1117:196–208.

19 Rodan GA, Martin TJ: Therapeutic approaches to bone diseases. Science 2000;289:1508–1514.

20 Soma S, et al: Effects of continuous infusion of PTH on experimental tooth movement in rats. J Bone Miner Res 1999;14:546–554.

21 Li F, et al: Effect of parathyroid hormone on experimental tooth movement in rats. Am J Orthod Dentofacial Orthop 2013;144:523–532.

22 Soma S, et al: Local and chronic application of PTH accelerates tooth movement in rats. J Dent Res 2000;79:1717–1724.

23 Kawasaki K, Shimizu N: Effects of low-energy laser irradiation on bone remodeling during experimental tooth movement in rats. Lasers Surg Med 2000;26:282–291.

24 Huang H, Williams RC, Kyrkanides S: Accelerated orthodontic tooth movement: molecular mechanisms. Am J Orthod Dentofacial Orthop 2014;146:620–632.

25 Collins MK, Sinclair PM: The local use of vitamin D to increase the rate of orthodontic tooth movement. Am J Orthod Dentofacial Orthop 1988;94:278–284.

26 Takano-Yamamoto T, et al: The effect of local application of 1,25-dihydroxycholecalciferol on osteoclast numbers in orthodontically treated rats. J Dent Res 1992;71:53–59.

27 Kale S, et al: Comparison of the effects of 1,25-dihydroxycholecalciferol and prostaglandin E_2 on orthodontic tooth movement. Am J Orthod Dentofacial Orthop 2004;125:607–614.

28 Meng R, et al: Crosstalk between integrin alphavbeta3 and estrogen receptor-alpha is involved in thyroid hormone-induced proliferation in human lung carcinoma cells. PLoS One 2011;6:e27547.

29 Bartzela T, et al: Medication effects on the rate of orthodontic tooth movement: a systematic literature review. Am J Orthod Dentofacial Orthop 2009;135:16–26.

30 Varga F, et al: T_3 affects expression of collagen I and collagen cross-linking in bone cell cultures. Biochem Biophys Res Commun 2010;402:180–185.

31 Endo T, Kobayashi T: Excess TSH causes abnormal skeletal development in young mice with hypothyroidism via suppressive effects on the growth plate. Am J Physiol Endocrinol Metab 2013;305:E660–E666.

32 Cray JJ Jr, et al: Effects of thyroxine exposure on osteogenesis in mouse calvarial pre-osteoblasts. PLoS One 2013;8:e69067.

33 Shirazi M, Dehpour AR, Jafari F: The effect of thyroid hormone on orthodontic tooth movement in rats. J Clin Pediatr Dent 1999;23:259–264.

34 Verna C, Dalstra M, Melsen B: The rate and the type of orthodontic tooth movement are influenced by bone turnover in a rat model. Eur J Orthod 2000;22:343–352.

35 Midgett RJ, Shaye R, Fruge JF Jr: The effect of altered bone metabolism on orthodontic tooth movement. Am J Orthod 1981;80:256–262.

36 Goldie RS, King GJ: Root resorption and tooth movement in orthodontically treated, calcium-deficient, and lactating rats. Am J Orthod 1984;85:424–430.

37 Engstrom C, Granstrom G, Thilander B: Effect of orthodontic force on periodontal tissue metabolism. A histologic and biochemical study in normal and hypocalcemic young rats. Am J Orthod Dentofacial Orthop 1988;93:486–495.

38 Hashimoto F, et al: Administration of osteocalcin accelerates orthodontic tooth movement induced by a closed coil spring in rats. Eur J Orthod 2001;23:535–545.

39 Hauschka PV, Lian JB, Gallop PM: Direct identification of the calcium-binding amino acid, gamma-carboxyglutamate, in mineralized tissue. Proc Natl Acad Sci U S A 1975;72:3925–3929.

40 Price RR, et al: Proceedings: regional and whole-body bone mineral content measurement with a rectilinear scanner. AJR Am J Roentgenol 1976;126:1277–1278.

41 Poser JW, et al: Isolation and sequence of the vitamin K-dependent protein from human bone. Undercarboxylation of the first glutamic acid residue. J Biol Chem 1980;255:8685–8691.

42 Ducy P, et al: Increased bone formation in osteocalcin-deficient mice. Nature 1996;382:448–452.

43 DeFranco DJ, et al: Normal bone particles are preferentially resorbed in the presence of osteocalcin-deficient bone particles in vivo. Calcif Tissue Int 1991;49:43–50.

44 Glowacki J, Lian JB: Impaired recruitment and differentiation of osteoclast progenitors by osteocalcin-deplete bone implants. Cell Differ 1987;21:247–254.

45 Chenu C, et al: Osteocalcin induces chemotaxis, secretion of matrix proteins, and calcium-mediated intracellular signaling in human osteoclast-like cells. J Cell Biol 1994;127:1149–1158.

46 Kobayashi Y, et al: Effects of local administration of osteocalcin on experimental tooth movement. Angle Orthod 1998;68:259–266.

47 Brooks PJ, et al: Molecular markers of early orthodontic tooth movement. Angle Orthod 2009;79:1108–1113.

48 Gustafson GT, Eckerdal O, Leever DL, Shanfeld JL, Montgomery P, Davidovitch Z: Cyclic AMP in dental and periodontal tissues during tooth eruption in kittens. J Dent Res 1977;56:407–415.

49 Leiker BJ, et al: The effects of exogenous prostaglandins on orthodontic tooth movement in rats. Am J Orthod Dentofacial Orthop 1995;108:380–388.

50 Seifi M, Eslami B, Saffar AS: The effect of prostaglandin E$_2$ and calcium gluconate on orthodontic tooth movement and root resorption in rats. Eur J Orthod 2003;25:199–204.

51 Sekhavat AR, et al: Effect of misoprostol, a prostaglandin E$_1$ analog, on orthodontic tooth movement in rats. Am J Orthod Dentofacial Orthop 2002;122:542–547.

52 Yamasaki K, Shibata Y, Fukuhara T: The effect of prostaglandins on experimental tooth movement in monkeys (Macaca fuscata). J Dent Res 1982;61:1444–1446.

53 Gurton AU, et al: Effects of PGI$_2$ and TxA$_2$ analogs and inhibitors in orthodontic tooth movement. Angle Orthod 2004;74:526–532.

54 Yamasaki K, et al: Clinical application of prostaglandin E$_1$ (PGE$_1$) upon orthodontic tooth movement. Am J Orthod 1984;85:508–518.

55 Walker JB, Buring SM: NSAID impairment of orthodontic tooth movement. Ann Pharmacother 2001;35:113–115.

56 Arias OR, Marquez-Orozco MC: Aspirin, acetaminophen, and ibuprofen: their effects on orthodontic tooth movement. Am J Orthod Dentofacial Orthop 2006;130:364–370.

57 Brudvik P, Rygh P: Root resorption after local injection of prostaglandin E$_2$ during experimental tooth movement. Eur J Orthod 1991;13:255–263.

58 Yamaguchi M, Kasai K: Inflammation in periodontal tissues in response to mechanical forces. Arch Immunol Ther Exp (Warsz) 2005;53:388–398.

59 Blessing M, Schirmacher P, Kaiser S: Overexpression of bone morphogenetic protein-6 (BMP-6) in the epidermis of transgenic mice: inhibition or stimulation of proliferation depending on the pattern of transgene expression and formation of psoriatic lesions. J Cell Biol 1996;135:227–239.

60 Andrade I Jr, Sousa AB, da Silva GG: New therapeutic modalities to modulate orthodontic tooth movement. Dental Press J Orthod 2014;19:123–133.

61 Drugarin D, Drugarin M, Negru S, Cioace R: RANK-RANKL/OPG molecular complex – control factors in bone remodeling. TMJ 2003;53:296–302.

62 Oshiro T, et al: Osteoclast induction in periodontal tissue during experimental movement of incisors in osteoprotegerin-deficient mice. Anat Rec 2002;266:218–225.

63 Kanzaki H, et al: Local RANKL gene transfer to the periodontal tissue accelerates orthodontic tooth movement. Gene Ther 2006;13:678–685.

64 Iglesias-Linares A, et al: The use of gene therapy vs corticotomy surgery in accelerating orthodontic tooth movement. Orthod Craniofac Res 2011;14:138–148.

65 Nicozisis JL, Nah-Cederquist HD, Tuncay OC: Relaxin affects the dentofacial sutural tissues. Clin Orthod Res 2000;3:192–201.

66 Madan MS, et al: Effects of human relaxin on orthodontic tooth movement and periodontal ligaments in rats. Am J Orthod Dentofacial Orthop 2007;131:8.e1–e10.

67 Liu ZJ, et al: Does human relaxin accelerate orthodontic tooth movement in rats? Ann N Y Acad Sci 2005;1041:388–394.

68 McGorray SP, et al: A randomized, placebo-controlled clinical trial on the effects of recombinant human relaxin on tooth movement and short-term stability. Am J Orthod Dentofacial Orthop 2012;141:196–203.

69 Matsuda N, et al: Role of epidermal growth factor and its receptor in mechanical stress-induced differentiation of human periodontal ligament cells in vitro. Arch Oral Biol 1998;43:987–997.

70 Kikuiri T, et al: Cyclic tension force activates nitric oxide production in cultured human periodontal ligament cells. J Periodontol 2000;71:533–539.

71 Nishimura M, et al: Periodontal tissue activation by vibration: intermittent stimulation by resonance vibration accelerates experimental tooth movement in rats. Am J Orthod Dentofacial Orthop 2008;133:572–583.

72 Ohmae M, Saito S, Morohashi T, Qu H, Seki K, Kurabayashi H, et al: Biomechanical acceleration of experimental tooth movement by ultrasonic vibration in vivo. 1. Homo-directional application of ultrasonication to orthodontic force. Orthod Waves 2001;60:201–212.

73 Trenter SC, Landini G, Walmsley AD: Effect of loading on the vibration characteristics of thin magnetostrictive ultrasonic scaler inserts. J Periodontol 2003;74:1308–1315.

74 Kau CH: A radiographic analysis of tooth morphology following the use of a novel cyclical force device in orthodontics. Head Face Med 2011;7:14.

75 Fukada E, Yasuda I: On the piezoelectric effect of bone. J Phys Soc Japan 1957;12:1158–1162.

76 Friedenberg ZB, et al: Bone reaction to varying amounts of direct current. Surg Gynecol Obstet 1970;131:894–899.

77 Davidovitch Z, et al: Electric currents, bone remodeling, and orthodontic tooth movement. II. Increase in rate of tooth movement and periodontal cyclic nucleotide levels by combined force and electric current. Am J Orthod 1980;77:33–47.

78 Hashimoto H: Effect of micro-pulsed electricity on experimental tooth movement. Nihon Kyosei Shika Gakkai Zasshi 1990;49:352–361.

79 Kim D-H, Park Y-G, Kang S-G: The effects of electrical current from a micro-electrical device on tooth movement. Korean J Orthod 2008;5:337–346.

80 Abdallah MN, Flores-Mir C: Are interventions for accelerating orthodontic tooth movement effective? Evid Based Dent 2014;15:116–117.

81 Camacho AD, Velasquez Cujar SA: Dental movement acceleration: literature review by an alternative scientific evidence method. World J Methodol 2014;4:151–162.

82 Darendeliler MA, Sinclair PM, Kusy RP: The effects of samarium-cobalt magnets and pulsed electromagnetic fields on tooth movement. Am J Orthod Dentofacial Orthop 1995;107:578–588.

83 Sakata M, et al: The effects of a static magnetic field on orthodontic tooth movement. J Orthod 2008;35:249–254.

84 Stark TM, Sinclair PM: Effect of pulsed electromagnetic fields on orthodontic tooth movement. Am J Orthod Dentofacial Orthop 1987;91:91–104.

85 Chen Q: Effect of pulsed electromagnetic field on orthodontic tooth movement through transmission electromicroscopy (in Chinese). Zhonghua Kou Qiang Yi Xue Za Zhi 1991;26:7–10, 61.

86 Showkatbakhsh R, Jamilian A, Showkatbakhsh M: The effect of pulsed electromagnetic fields on the acceleration of tooth movement. World J Orthod 2010;11:e52–e56.

87 Tengku BS, et al: Effect of a static magnetic field on orthodontic tooth movement in the rat. Eur J Orthod 2000;22:475–487.

88 Kolahi J, Abrishami M, Davidovitch Z: Microfabricated biocatalytic fuel cells: a new approach to accelerating the orthodontic tooth movement. Med Hypotheses 2009;73:340–341.

89 Mester E, Mester AF, Mester A: The biomedical effects of laser application. Lasers Surg Med 1985;5:31–39.

90 Soudry M, et al: Effect of a helium-neon laser on cellular growth: an in vitro study of human gingival fibroblasts (in French). J Biol Buccale 1988;16:129–135.

91 Schultz RJ, et al: Effects of varying intensities of laser energy on articular cartilage: a preliminary study. Lasers Surg Med 1985;5:577–588.

92 Balboni GC, et al: Effect of laser irradiation on collagen production by fibroblasts in vitro (in French). Bull Assoc Anat (Nancy) 1985;69:15–18.

93 Anders JJ, et al: Low power laser irradiation alters the rate of regeneration of the rat facial nerve. Lasers Surg Med 1993;13:72–82.

94 Trelles MA, Mayayo E: Bone fracture consolidates faster with low-power laser. Lasers Surg Med 1987;7:36–45.

95 Lim HM, Lew KK, Tay DK: A clinical investigation of the efficacy of low level laser therapy in reducing orthodontic postadjustment pain. Am J Orthod Dentofacial Orthop 1995;108:614–622.

96 Rodrigues MTJ, Ribciro MS, Groth EB, Zezell DM: Evaluation of effects of laser therapy (λ = 830 nm) on oral ulceration induced by fixed orthodontic appliances. Lasers Surg Med 2002; 30(suppl 14):15.

97 Khadra M, et al: Enhancement of bone formation in rat calvarial bone defects using low-level laser therapy. Oral Surg Oral Med Oral Pathol Oral Radiol Endod 2004;97:693–700.

98 Conlan MJ, Rapley JW, Cobb CM: Biostimulation of wound healing by low-energy laser irradiation. A review. J Clin Periodontol 1996;23:492–496.

99 Saito S, Shimizu N: Stimulatory effects of low-power laser irradiation on bone regeneration in midpalatal suture during expansion in the rat. Am J Orthod Dentofacial Orthop 1997;111:525–532.

100 Sun X, et al: Effects of low energy laser on tooth movement and remodeling of alveolar bone in rabbits (in Chinese). Hua Xi Kou Qiang Yi Xue Za Zhi 2001; 19:290–293.

101 Goulart CS, et al: Photoradiation and orthodontic movement: experimental study with canines. Photomed Laser Surg 2006;24:192–196.

102 Yoshida T, et al: Low-energy laser irradiation accelerates the velocity of tooth movement via stimulation of the alveolar bone remodeling. Orthod Craniofac Res 2009;12:289–298.

103 Habib FA, et al: Laser-induced alveolar bone changes during orthodontic movement: a histological study on rodents. Photomed Laser Surg 2010;28: 823–830.

104 Fujita S, et al: Low-energy laser stimulates tooth movement velocity via expression of RANK and RANKL. Orthod Craniofac Res 2008;11:143–155.

105 Altan BA, et al: Metrical and histological investigation of the effects of low-level laser therapy on orthodontic tooth movement. Lasers Med Sci 2012; 27:131–140.

106 Yamaguchi M, et al: Low-energy laser irradiation facilitates the velocity of tooth movement and the expressions of matrix metalloproteinase-9, cathepsin K, alpha(v) beta(3) integrin in rats. Eur J Orthod 2010;32:131–139.

107 Katagiri T, Takahashi N: Regulatory mechanisms of osteoblast and osteoclast differentiation. Oral Dis 2002;8: 147–159.

108 Aihara N, Yamaguchi M, Kasai K: Low-energy irradiation stimulates formation of osteoclast-like cells via RANK expression in vitro. Lasers Med Sci 2006;21:24–33.

109 Zhu X, Chen Y, Sun X: A study on expression of basic fibroblast growth factors in periodontal tissue following orthodontic tooth movement associated with low power laser irradiation (in Chinese). Hua Xi Kou Qiang Yi Xue Za Zhi 2002;20:166–168.

110 Limpanichkul W, et al: Effects of low-level laser therapy on the rate of orthodontic tooth movement. Orthod Craniofac Res 2006;9:38–43.

111 Gama SK, Habib FA, Monteiro JS, Paraguassú GM, Araújo TM, Cangussú MC, Pinheiro AL: Tooth movement after infrared laser phototherapy: clinical study in rodents. Photomed Laser Surg 2010;28(suppl 2):79–83.

112 Cruz DR, et al: Effects of low-intensity laser therapy on the orthodontic movement velocity of human teeth: a preliminary study. Lasers Surg Med 2004; 35:117–120.

113 Youssef M, et al: The effect of low-level laser therapy during orthodontic movement: a preliminary study. Lasers Med Sci 2008;23:27–33.

114 Sousa MV, et al: Influence of low-level laser on the speed of orthodontic movement. Photomed Laser Surg 2011;29:191–196.

115 Genc G, et al: Effect of low-level laser therapy (LLLT) on orthodontic tooth movement. Lasers Med Sci 2013;28: 41–47.

116 Kau CH: Biotechnology in orthodontics photo biomodulation. Dentistry 2012;2:e108.

117 Oron U, et al: Ga-As (808 nm) laser irradiation enhances ATP production in human neuronal cells in culture. Photomed Laser Surg 2007;25:180–182.

118 Kau CH, et al: Photobiomodulation accelerates orthodontic alignment in the early phase of treatment. Prog Orthod 2013;14:30.

119 Tuby H, Maltz L, Oron U: Low-level laser irradiation (LLLI) promotes proliferation of mesenchymal and cardiac stem cells in culture. Lasers Surg Med 2007;39:373–378.

120 Vinck EM, Cagnie BJ, Cornelissen MJ, Declercq HA, Cambier DC: Increased fibroblast proliferation induced by light emitting diode and low power laser irradiation. Lasers Med Sci 2003; 18:95–99.

121 Doshi-Mehta G, Bhad-Patil WA: Efficacy of low-intensity laser therapy in reducing treatment time and orthodontic pain: a clinical investigation. Am J Orthod Dentofacial Orthop 2012; 141:289–297.

122 Kau CH: Orthodontics in the 21st century: a view from across the pond. J Orthod 2012;39:75–76.

123 Ekizer A, et al: Effect of LED-mediated-photobiomodulation therapy on orthodontic tooth movement and root resorption in rats. Lasers Med Sci 2015;30:779–785.

Alpdogan Kantarci, DDS, PhD
Forsyth Institute
245 First Street
Cambridge, MA 02142 (USA)
E-Mail akantarci@forsyth.org

Kantarci A, Will L, Yen S (eds): Tooth Movement. Front Oral Biol. Basel, Karger, 2016, vol 18, pp 92–101
DOI: 10.1159/000382051

Surgical Methods for the Acceleration of the Orthodontic Tooth Movement

Konstantinia Almpani · Alpdogan Kantarci

Forsyth Institute, Cambridge, Mass., USA

Abstract

Surgical techniques for the acceleration of the orthodontic tooth movement have been tested for more than 100 years in clinical practice. Since original methods have been extremely invasive and have been associated with increased tooth morbidity and various other gaps, the research in this field has always followed an episodic trend. Modern approaches represent a well-refined strategy where the concept of the bony block has been abandoned and only a cortical plate around the orthodontic tooth movement has been desired. Selective alveolar decortication has been a reproducible gold standard to this end. Its proposed mechanism has been the induction of rapid orthodontic tooth movement through the involvement of the periodontal ligament. More recent techniques included further refinement of this procedure through less invasive techniques such as the use of piezo-electricity and corticision. This chapter focuses on the evolution of the surgical approaches and the mechanistic concepts underlying the biological process during the surgically accelerated orthodontic tooth movement.

Orthodontics has been developing greatly in achieving the desired results, both clinically and technically. Computer software-aided treatment planning, 3-dimensional cephalometric analysis and assessment, continuous modifications and improvement in the field of biomaterials and bioengineering and the automated fabrication of individualized fixed appliances have greatly improved the biomechanical efficiency of orthodontic treatment. Consequently, treatment time quality and duration have greatly improved.

However, the average active orthodontic treatment duration with a significant variation, which can be influenced by several factors [1, 2], is 1–2 years. This is still considered a relatively long treatment time duration for a patient to be committed to. A long follow-up retention period is normally added to that period. Therefore, there has been a continuous search for methods to enhance the rate and efficacy of orthodontic tooth movement. Attempts to accelerate tooth movement can be dated back to the 1890s, almost contemporary with Angle's groundbreaking work in modern orthodontics [3]. Over the years, several case reports, narrative reviews and clinical research papers have discussed various aspects of techniques used for accelerated orthodontic tooth movement.

Orthodontic tooth movement depends on the modeling and remodeling processes of the alveolar bone that take place in response to mechanical forces and which determine the quantity and quality of orthodontic tooth movement [4]. The rate of alveolar modeling and remodeling is determined by the level of activity of bone cells (osteoclasts, osteoblasts and osteocytes), which are under the control of mechanical and biochemical factors. A number of techniques have been introduced to accelerate orthodontic tooth movement, by interfering with many of the above mechanisms and biological paths. These techniques can be briefly categorized as surgical and nonsurgical.

Acceleration of orthodontic movement is important for both clinicians and orthodontic patients. Apart from the obvious benefit of shorter total treatment duration, there is a number of concomitant equally significant advantages. A reduction in treatment duration simultaneously contributes in the direct decrease in the rates of time-dependent unwanted side effects, such as oral-hygiene-related problems, root resorption and open gingival embrasure spaces [5–9]. Moreover, tooth movement enhancement in most cases has an additional positive impact not only on the speed, but also on the rate of tooth movement, expanding the envelope of tooth movement even further. Differential tooth movement might also become much easier, and posttreatment stability has been proven to become significantly improved, as a result of increased bone turnover.

Adult patients, in particular, are the ones that could mostly benefit by the advances in this field. The reason is that adult orthodontic patients normally have more specific objectives and concerns related to facial and dental aesthetics, the type of orthodontic appliances and the duration of treatment or need the treatment as part of a more complicated interdisciplinary treatment plan. Biologically-wise, there is no growth to take advantage of, and local tissue metabolism and regeneration rates are much lower in comparison to adolescents and children. Finally, adult patients are more prone to periodontal complications [10].

The aim of this chapter is to present the historical background and the contemporary surgical techniques that have been investigated for the purpose of tooth movement acceleration. Surgical techniques that have been tested include alveolar osteotomy- and/or alveolar corticotomy-assisted tooth movement, distraction osteogenesis-assisted tooth movement procedures, interseptal bone reduction, orthognathic 'surgery-first' orthodontic treatment and fiberotomy. Some of these interventions have never become popularized, because of the invasiveness of their nature and potent surgical side effects. However, their effects have been repeatedly reported to significantly increase the rate of orthodontic tooth movement, and many of these techniques are still a subject of many investigations, mainly the concept of interdisciplinary treatment cases. Orthodontic tooth movement, in these cases, can synchronize with tissue-engineering principles of periodontal regenerative surgery in order to create rapid orthodontic movement and overcome its side effects [11].

Alveolar Osteotomy-Assisted Tooth Movement

Osteotomy is defined as a surgical cut through both the cortical and trabecular bones. This term is frequently used when describing the creation of bone segments. Corticotomy, on the other hand, is a surgical cut where only the cortical bone is involved, perforated or mechanically altered in a controlled surgical manner [12].

In orthodontics, osteotomies have been used to enhance and accelerate tooth movement. In 1893, Cunningham presented 'Luxation, or the immediate method in the treatment of irregular teeth' at the International Dental Congress in Chicago. He used mesial and distal interseptal osteotomies to reposition palatally inclined maxillary teeth and stabilized them in correct occlusion with wire ligatures or metal splints. The most important feature was the fact that this combined active surgical-orthodontic treatment reduced the procedure time to one third that of conventional treatment and allowed more predictable treatment in older patients [13]. About 50 years later, Bichlmayr was the first to use the corticotomy procedure for the closure of diastemata in patients over 16 years old, in maxillary incisor protrusion cases treated with first premolar extractions. This procedure involved division of the palatal cortex overlying the incisors, and excision of alveolar bone distal to the canines, in order to speed up the whole treatment process [13].

In the 1950s, Köle [14] introduced his 'bony block' technique, a surgical procedure involving both osteotomy and corticotomy to accelerate orthodontic tooth movement, based on the concept that teeth move faster when the resistance exerted by the surrounding cortical bone is reduced via a surgical procedure. Köle further explained that the reduced resistance enhances an en bloc movement of the entire alveolar cortical segment, which is connected by softer medullary bone including the confined teeth, when exposed to orthodontic forces. Köle's procedure involves the reflection of full thickness flaps to expose buccal and lingual alveolar bone, followed by interdental cuts through the cortical bone, barely penetrating the medullary bone [15]. This theory of en bloc movement to enhance tooth movement prevailed in several subsequent reports [16–20].

These initial approaches included some types of alveolar osteotomy alone or combined with corticotomy. Traditionally, vertical and horizontal osteotomies have had an increased risk of postoperative tooth devitalization or even bone necrosis, depending on the severity of injury to the trabecular bone [13]. There is also an increased risk of periodontal damage, mainly in cases in which the interradicular space is less than 2 mm [21].

Alveolar Corticotomy-Assisted Tooth Movement

Alveolar corticotomies are defined as the surgical interventions where the incision must pierce the cortical layer and, at the same time, penetrate into the bone marrow only minimally [22]. The invasiveness of the corticotomy procedures requiring full mucoperiosteal flaps constituted a serious drawback for their widespread acceptance among orthodontists and patients. Therefore, more conservative flapless corticotomy-restricted techniques have recently been proposed [19, 23]. These procedures can be completed more quickly and might be preferable if patient discomfort is indeed minimized and if treatment efficiency is maintained. Corticotomy has many advantages compared with osteotomy. It prevents injuries of the periodontium, pocket formation and devitalizing of the adjacent teeth. The nutritive function of the bone is also maintained through the spongiosa avoiding the possibility of aseptic bone necrosis [14].

Despite the evolution of clinical methods, the scientific explanation of accelerated tooth movement was still believed, until recently, to be a reduced mechanical resistance after osteotomy or corticotomy, enabling the teeth to be moved en bloc with the tissues surrounding them [17–20, 22, 24, 25]. This view was challenged by Wilcko et al. [26, 27]. They described an innovative strategy of combining corticotomy alveolar surgery with alveolar grafting in a technique referred to, initially, as accelerated osteogenic orthodontics and, more recently, as periodontally accelerated osteogenic orthodontics.

Wilcko's technique combines fixed orthodontic appliances, labial and palatal/lingual corticotomies, and bone grafting with demineralized freeze-dried bone and bovine bone with clindamycin. This procedure involving corticotomy with subsequent bone augmentation has been proposed to increase the volume of the alveolar process, to facilitate arch development, to prevent or even treat fenestrations, and to maximize the metabolic response during orthodontic treatment. Tooth movement can be initiated 2 weeks after surgery. They reported rapid tooth movement at a rate of 3–4 times greater than conventional orthodontic movement [26, 27]. Respectively, according to the results of the same studies, periodontally accelerated osteogenic orthodontics treatment can often be completed in one third to one fourth of the time required for traditional orthodontic treatment [28].

Wilcko et al. [26, 27] were first to suggest that tooth movement assisted with corticotomy may be due to a demineralization-remineralization process rather than bony block movement. This process resembled the regional acceleratory phenomenon (RAP), a term initially used to describe rare cases of accelerated fracture healing [29]. It is indeed an exaggerated response from that organism to an injured area to facilitate healing and has been associated with local increased bone turnover and decreased bone density. The tissue response varies in duration, size and intensity, depending on the magnitude of the stimulus [29].

However, the RAP in the case of orthodontic tooth movement has also been attributed to the increased chemoattraction of macrophages. These macrophages remove the hyaline zone within 1 week after the application of orthodontic force [30, 31]. This early disappearance of the hyaline zone results in the acceleration of the tooth movement process around the corticotomy alveolar area. Thus, the RAP is influenced by both bone density and the degree of hyalinization of the periodontal ligament [4, 32–34].

The literature confirms the fact that corticotomies induce an RAP reaction that has an acceleratory effect on orthodontic movement. A variety of animal studies has been conducted in order to better understand the biological effects of corticotomies on orthodontic tooth movement [20, 30, 31, 35–42]. The results of the above studies are relatively uniform in showing that the rate of tooth movement is accelerated on corticotomy-treated dentoalveolar areas, in comparison to untreated control sides or groups. The amount of movement in most of the studies was doubled over the time of corticotomy-assisted treatment at the rate of about 1 mm/month [31, 36, 37, 39]. However, the duration of the RAP event was limited.

Numerous corticotomy-assisted orthodontic case reports have also been published, with encouragingly positive results. Corticotomy procedures have been reported to significantly accelerate orthodontic molar intrusion [43–45], distalization [46] and maxillary arch expansion [26]. There are also case studies reporting a reduction in total orthodontic treatment duration with the aid of alveolar corticotomy. In specific, full cases involving resolution of crowding [47, 48], skeletal class II division 2 correction [47], retraction of mandibular incisors [49], extraction cases [30] and anterior open bite correction [50] were completed in as little as 6–19 months. Respectively, prospective clinical studies have also reported faster tooth movement [51–53] and completion of treatment [38], with the use of alveolar corticotomies.

The duration of the RAP usually lasts about 4–6 months in human bone, before it returns to a normal turnover rate [54]. Therefore, this phenomenon gives to the orthodontist a 'window' period of at least 4 months for accelerated movement [52, 55]. During this period, corticotomy-facilitated teeth moved on average twice faster than the control side. The degree to which corticotomies might be expected to reduce the overall treatment duration depends on the type of treatment required and is yet to be defined.

A number of different corticotomy variations have been tested, such as alveolar interseptal corticotomy [56], selective alveolar decortication [37] and interseptal bone reduction [57]. The outcomes of these experiments also indicated that the rate of tooth movement was significantly increased on the corticotomy-treated sites. No associated side effects like increased root resorption or irreversible pulp injuries have been reported so far, although the currently existing evidence is considered as inadequate.

Recently, Kim et al. [41] also introduced the 'corticision' technique as a minimally invasive alternative to corticotomy, creating a surgical injury to the bone without flap reflection. In this technique, a reinforced scalpel and a mallet were used in order to access the cortical bone, without raising flaps. This surgical injury was evaluated as adequate to induce the RAP effect and make the teeth move more rapidly during orthodontic treatment. This technique, although innovative, has a few major drawbacks: the inability to graft soft or hard tissues during the procedure to correct osseous and soft tissue deficiencies and reinforce the periodontium, and, in some cases, transient postsurgical dizziness from the repeated malleting during the surgery.

In the same year, Keser and Dibart [58] proposed a new and minimally invasive procedure that they named 'piezocision'. Like periodontally accelerated osteogenic orthodontics, it also speeds up tooth movement by alveolar corticotomy, but instead of full-thickness flaps, small vertical cuts through the gingival tissues and periosteum are made to reach the bone cortex. Bone grafts are embedded in tunnels connecting the vertical cuts. According to case reports in the literature, it appears that piezocision is similarly effective in accelerating tooth movement and augmenting periodontal tissues with much less trauma [58–60].

'Piezopuncture' is another minimally invasive novel perio-orthodontic technique, which enables rapid orthodontic movement. This technique involves puncturing of the cortical bone with a piezosurgical regimen, which induces a local RAP response. This procedure has only been tested in dogs. Further studies on the optimal power range of a piezosurgical device to induce

an RAP with orthodontic tooth movement are suggested for secure clinical applications [61]. In addition, Vercellotti and Podesta [62] proposed the use of a piezoelectric knife instead of a high-speed surgical bur in order to decrease the surgical trauma. Because of its micrometric and selective cut, a piezoelectric device produces safe and precise osteotomies without osteonecrotic damage [63, 64]. Nevertheless, more studies are needed about the mechanisms of piezocision to accelerate tooth movement and to evaluate its effectiveness and long-term results.

For the orthodontist, the combination of minor surgery and enhanced orthodontic tooth movement is intriguing. However, despite the fact that the corticotomy technique and its variations have been proved to be quite effective in accelerating tooth movement, there are still several obstacles preventing its more widespread use. Surgical complications associated mainly with extensive corticotomy sites, such as postoperative pain and swelling [15] and subcutaneous hematomas of the face and neck [18, 65], have been reported and may negatively impact the patients' experiences and acceptance rate of the procedure.

In addition, the duration of the RAP is limited in comparison to the total treatment duration. Thus, although alveolar corticotomy might have proven to be effective in accelerating tooth movement by different studies, it is not fair to form any conclusions regarding its effect on the overall treatment duration, without evaluating the quality of the results [66]. Finally, even though there is generally no need for costly additional equipment, the additional cost to orthodontic treatment to cover the surgical procedures can also be a concern [67].

Distraction Osteogenesis

Distraction osteogenesis is a method for generating new bone by progressively distracting healing surfaces, following the complete osteotomy of a bone. Essentially it is a bone-modeling procedure that produces perivascular woven bone, which then condenses and remodels to mature lamellar bone [68]. It is suggested that formation of new bone with a width of approximately 1 mm/day can be achieved by this method [69].

Distraction osteogenesis was used as early as 1904 by Codivilla [70] and was later popularized by the clinical and research studies of Ilizarov in Russia. Distraction osteogenesis was performed in the human mandible by Guerrero [71] in 1990 and McCarthy et al. [72] in 1992. Various indications in the oral and maxillofacial region have been subsequently described [72–74].

Liou and Huang [75] were the first to apply this concept to orthodontic tooth movement in order to perform rapid canine retraction through distraction osteogenesis of the periodontal ligament. They considered the periodontal ligament as a 'suture' between alveolar bone and tooth and investigated the accelerated orthodontic tooth movement into newly distracted bone after mandibular distraction osteogenesis in a canine model in humans. Their results showed that rapid orthodontic tooth movement can be achieved with this technique.

In a more recent study, Sayin et al. [76] investigated the clinical validation of the original technique of Liou and Huang in another prospective clinical study, confirming that tooth movement via distraction of the periodontal ligament significantly reduces the treatment time. Sukurica et al. [77] also achieved rapid canine retraction in a number of patients performing osteotomies surrounding the teeth in the dentoalveolar segment, in compliance with the principles of distraction osteogenesis.

Kişnişci et al. [78] and Işeri et al. [79] presented a different technique for rapid canine distalization by performing osteotomies surrounding the canines and also achieved rapid movement of the canines in the dentoalveolar segment, in compliance with the principles of distraction osteogenesis. They named this technique dentoalveolar distraction. According to their studies, the dentoalveolar distraction technique reduces orthodontic treatment duration by 6–9 months in patients who need extraction, with no need for extraoral or intraoral anchorage devices and with not unfavorable short-term effects in the periodontal tissues and surrounding structures [78, 79]. Other clinical researchers seem to agree with their results [80].

No evidence of complications such as root fracture, root resorption, ankylosis or serious soft tissue dehiscences was reported in any of these studies at the end of dentoalveolar distraction, at least in the short term. However, a number of other complications have been associated with the distraction osteogenesis techniques, such as increase in gingival sulcus depth [77], anchorage loss [76], tipping of the anchorage and retracted teeth [75, 77] and, more frequently, loss of pulpal vitality [75, 77].

Currently, the available distractors are bulky, unidirectional and unavailable on the market. They need to be refined, developed and oriented with fixed appliances in the future. Moreover, the long-term effects of this method are unknown, and histological research is needed.

Orthognathic 'Surgery-First' Treatment

Orthodontists have long noted increased rates of tooth movement following orthognathic surgical procedures [68]. This effect is usually attributed to a postoperative RAP phenomenon, stimulated by the wound healing of the surgical areas [81, 82]. Traditional comprehensive orthodontic/orthognathic surgery treatment starts with orthodontic treatment that usually aligns and decompensates the teeth in each dental arch independently, as a preparation stage for the following optimum surgical correction of the skeletal discrepancies. After surgery, orthodontic treatment is normally required in order to achieve optimum occlusal relationships. Typically, the total treatment time is about 24–30 months.

Surgery-first orthodontics is a strategy that significantly shortens treatment duration for patients who need orthognathic surgery, by taking advantage of the generalized RAP osseous effect [81, 83–89]. In addition, the quality of treatment, based on facial esthetics, dental occlusion and stability of the results, is equally satisfactory. Moreover, dental occlusion and facial esthetics usually show immediate improvement after surgery, which is very positive for the patient's psychology and cooperation. This is a fact that has to be seriously considered in the treatment planning of orthognathic surgery cases. Nevertheless, careful patient selection, precise treatment planning and clinical experience by both the surgeon and the orthodontist in the field of orthognathic surgery are required [87, 89].

Fiberotomy

Fiberotomy is the surgical detachment of the marginal gingivae from the root surface and therefore separation of the mucoperiosteum from the alveolar bone. According to past and more recent studies in animals, fiberotomy alone may also accelerate orthodontic tooth movement to a certain degree [38, 54, 90, 91].

This kind of incision seems to cause an abrupt drop of cellular strains of gingival fibroblasts [90], activating a chain of signals that propagate osteoclastogenic alveolar bone resorption on its periodontal ligament surfaces of the alveolar bone. Detachment of the mucoperiosteum from bone surfaces also yields a direct mild burst of local bone remodeling on its outer surfaces, which has been characterized as an RAP effect [29, 90]. Consequently, increased local bone turnover has as a result the acceleration of orthodontic tooth movement of the adjacent teeth.

Conclusions

Overall, the results from the application of different surgical techniques indicate that acceleration of tooth movement to a clinically significant rate is indeed possible. Surgical techniques could be really helpful in interdisciplinary treatment cases, where dental extraction and/or periodontal surgery are required for other reasons. There has been a lot of consistency in the positive results of accelerated corticotomy-assisted tooth movement. Flapless and minimally invasive methods are certainly more attractive, for the decrease in possible side effects. Finally, case selection and detailed interdisciplinary treatment planning are very important for surgical interventions, considering their time-dependent effect in orthodontic movement acceleration.

According to the results of recently published systematic reviews and meta-analyses, the highest level of evidence for accelerating orthodontic dental movement procedures is for 'surgery-first' orthodontic cases, followed by corticotomy and low-level laser application. Nevertheless, the results of the relative studies should be interpreted with caution given the small number, quality and heterogeneity of the exciting data [92–95].

At present, further research and more randomized high-quality studies in humans are required, in order to be able to confirm the claimed advantages of the currently investigated techniques and to be able to evaluate their effects, not only in the duration, but also in the quality of treatment. Moreover, additional effort should be made for the formation of specific protocols, more thorough reporting on possible adverse effects, longer follow-up periods, cost-benefit analyses and total treatment duration effect evaluation.

Finally, more research is also required at a molecular level. It is essential to fully understand the molecular mechanisms underlying the process of accelerated orthodontic tooth movement. This knowledge would be extremely valuable for the evolution of the existing procedures and/or the development of new techniques that would be even more efficient, with minimal side effects and with the lowest cost. New knowledge in this field will empower us to revolutionize orthodontic therapy and its practice in the future.

References

1 Mavreas D, Athanasiou AE: Factors affecting the duration of orthodontic treatment: a systematic review. Eur J Orthod 2008;30:386–395.

2 Fisher MA, Wenger RM, Hans MG: Pretreatment characteristics associated with orthodontic treatment duration. Am J Orthod Dentofacial Orthop 2010; 137:178–186.

3 Fitzpatrick BN: Corticotomy. Aust Dent J 1980;25:255–258.

4 Verna C, Dalstra M, Melsen B: The rate and the type of orthodontic tooth movement is influenced by bone turnover in a rat model. Eur J Orthod 2000;22:343–352.

5 Brin I, et al: External apical root resorption in class II malocclusion: a retrospective review of 1- versus 2-phase treatment. Am J Orthod Dentofacial Orthop 2003;124:151–156.

6 Sunku R, et al: Quantitative digital subtraction radiography in the assessment of external apical root resorption induced by orthodontic therapy: a retrospective study. J Contemp Dent Pract 2011;12:422–428.

7 Jiang RP, McDonald JP, Fu MK: Root resorption before and after orthodontic treatment: a clinical study of contributory factors. Eur J Orthod 2010;32:693–697.

8 Richter AE, et al: Incidence of caries lesions among patients treated with comprehensive orthodontics. Am J Orthod Dentofacial Orthop 2011;139:657–664.

9 Ikeda T, et al: Prediction and causes of open gingival embrasure spaces between the mandibular central incisors following orthodontic treatment. Aust Orthod J 2004;20:87–92.

10 Ong MM, Wang HL: Periodontic and orthodontic treatment in adults. Am J Orthod Dentofacial Orthop 2002;122: 420–428.

11 Little RM: Stability and relapse of dental arch alignment; in Burstone CJ, Nanda R (eds): Retention and Stability in Orthodontics. Philadelphia, Saunders, 1993, pp 97–106.

12 Murphy NC, Wilcko MT, Bissada NF, Davidovitch Z, Enlow DH, Dashe J: Corticotomy-facilitated orthodontics: clarion call or siren song; in Brugnami F, Caiazzo A (eds): Orthodontically Driven Corticotomy: Tissue Engineering to Enhance Orthodontic and Multidisciplinary Treatment. Hoboken, Wiley-Blackwell, 2014, pp 1–39.

13 Cano J, et al: Corticotomy-assisted orthodontics. J Clin Exp Dent 2012;4:e54–e59.

14 Köle H: Surgical operations on the alveolar ridge to correct occlusal abnormalities. Oral Surg Oral Med Oral Pathol 1959;12:515–529.

15 Amit G, et al: Periodontally accelerated osteogenic orthodontics (PAOO) – a review. J Clin Exp Dent 2012;4:e292–e296.

16 Bell WH, Levy BM: Revascularization and bone healing after maxillary corticotomies. J Oral Surg 1972;30:218–226.

17 Anholm JM, et al: Corticotomy-facilitated orthodontics. CDA J 1986;14:7–11.

18 Gantes B, Rathbun E, Anholm M: Effects on the periodontium following corticotomy-facilitated orthodontics. Case reports. J Periodontol 1990;61:234–238.

19 Suya H: Corticotomy in orthodontics; in Hosl E, Baldauf A (eds): Mechanical and Biological Basics in Orthodontic Therapy. Heidelberg, Hütlig, 1991, pp 207–226.

20 Duker J: Experimental animal research into segmental alveolar movement after corticotomy. J Maxillofac Surg 1975;3: 81–84.

21 Merrill RG, Pedersen GW: Interdental osteotomy for immediate repositioning of dental-osseous elements. J Oral Surg 1976;34:118–125.

22 Chung KR, Oh MY, Ko SJ: Corticotomy-assisted orthodontics. J Clin Orthod 2001;35:331–339.

23 Roblee RD, Bolding SL, Landers JM: Surgically facilitated orthodontic therapy: a new tool for optimal interdisciplinary results. Compend Contin Educ Dent 2009;30:264–275; quiz 276–278.

24 Generson RM, et al: Combined surgical and orthodontic management of anterior open bite using corticotomy. J Oral Surg 1978;36:216–219.

25 Amimoto A, et al: Effects of surgical orthodontic treatment for malalignment due to the prolonged retention of deciduous canines in young dogs. J Vet Med Sci 1993;55:73–79.

26 Wilcko WM, et al: Rapid orthodontics with alveolar reshaping: two case reports of decrowding. Int J Periodontics Restorative Dent 2001;21:9–19.

27 Wilcko MT, et al: Accelerated osteogenic orthodontics technique: a 1-stage surgically facilitated rapid orthodontic technique with alveolar augmentation. J Oral Maxillofac Surg 2009;67:2149–2159.

28 Wilcko W, Wilcko MT: Accelerating tooth movement: the case for corticotomy-induced orthodontics. Am J Orthod Dentofacial Orthop 2013;144:4–12.

29 Frost HM: The biology of fracture healing. An overview for clinicians. Part I. Clin Orthop Relat Res 1989;248:283–293.

30 Iino S, Sakoda S, Miyawaki S: An adult bimaxillary protrusion treated with corticotomy-facilitated orthodontics and titanium miniplates. Angle Orthod 2006; 76:1074–1082.

31 Sanjideh PA, et al: Tooth movements in foxhounds after one or two alveolar corticotomies. Eur J Orthod 2010;32:106–113.

32 Verna C, Melsen B: Tissue reaction to orthodontic tooth movement in different bone turnover conditions. Orthod Craniofac Res 2003;6:155–163.

33 Goldie RS, King GJ: Root resorption and tooth movement in orthodontically treated, calcium-deficient, and lactating rats. Am J Orthod 1984;85:424–430.

34 Von Bohl M, et al: Focal hyalinization during experimental tooth movement in beagle dogs. Am J Orthod Dentofacial Orthop 2004;125:615–623.

35 Cho KW, et al: The effect of cortical activation on orthodontic tooth movement. Oral Dis 2007;13:314–319.

36 Iino S, et al: Acceleration of orthodontic tooth movement by alveolar corticotomy in the dog. Am J Orthod Dentofacial Orthop 2007;131:448.e1–e8.

37 Sebaoun JD, et al: Modeling of trabecular bone and lamina dura following selective alveolar decortication in rats. J Periodontol 2008;79:1679–1688.

38 Lee W, et al: Corticotomy-/osteotomy-assisted tooth movement microCTs differ. J Dent Res 2008;87:861–867.

Kantarci A, Will L, Yen S (eds): Tooth Movement. Front Oral Biol. Basel, Karger, 2016, vol 18, pp 102–108
DOI: 10.1159/000351903

Piezocision™: Accelerating Orthodontic Tooth Movement While Correcting Hard and Soft Tissue Deficiencies

Serge Dibart

Department of Periodontology and Oral Biology, Boston University Henry M. Goldman School of Dental Medicine, Boston, Mass., USA

Abstract

Piezocision™-assisted orthodontics is an innovative, minimally invasive surgical procedure designed to help achieve rapid orthodontic tooth movement while correcting/preventing mucogingival defects by adding bone and/or soft tissues. Microsurgical interproximal openings are done in the buccal gingiva to let the piezoelectric knife create the bone injury that will lead to transient demineralization and subsequent accelerated tooth movement. This technique can be used for the whole mouth, the cuts being simultaneously performed at the maxilla and the mandible (generalized Piezocision) or for segments of the dentition (localized Piezocision) to achieve specific localized results (intrusion, extrusion, distalization of teeth, etc.).

Surgical interventions on the alveolar ridges that are aimed at facilitating orthodontic treatment are not new [1]. Among the many procedures described in the literature, the work done by the Wilcko brothers on this subject stands out as seminal [2]. In their 2003 article, they report a case treated with alveolar decortications concomitant with bone grafting to expand alveolar volume and allow for rapid tooth movement into the newly expanded sites [3]. This approach combining a corticotomy-facilitated orthodontic treatment and periodontal alveolar augmentation has been named the accelerated osteogenic orthodontic procedure. It requires the elevation of buccal and lingual full thickness flaps, with extensive decortications of the buccal and lingual alveolar bone. This physical injury is responsible for the initiation of a temporary demineralization process coupled with an increased regional bone turnover that characterizes the regional acceleratory phenomenon (RAP) [4–6]. The authors surmised that this transient osteopenia (diminished bone density, same bone volume) is responsible for the rapid tooth movement, as the teeth move in a more 'pliable' environment. In 2007, Vercelotti and Podesta [7] introduced the use of piezosurgery in conjunction with the conventional flap elevations to create an environment conducive to rapid tooth movement. Although quite effective, these techniques are also quite invasive in nature as they require extensive flap elevations and osseous surgery. They have the potential to generate postsurgical discomfort as well as postoperative complications. Because of these shortcomings they have not been widely embraced by the patient or dental communities. Park et al. [8] in 2006 and Kim et al. [9] in 2009 introduced the corticision technique as a minimally invasive alternative to create surgical injury to the bone without flap reflection. In this technique, the authors use a reinforced scalpel and a mallet to go through the gingiva and cortical bone, without raising a flap bucally and lingually. The surgical injury created is enough to induce the RAP effect and move the teeth rapidly during orthodontic treatment. This technique, although innovative does not provide grafting of soft or hard tissues to correct anatomical inadequacies and reinforce the periodontium. In 2009, we introduced a new minimally invasive procedure that we called 'Piezocision™' [10]. This technique combines microincisions with selective tunneling that allows for hard or soft tissue grafting and piezoelectric bone decortication [11, 12].

Indications

- Class I malocclusions with moderate-to-severe crowding (nonextraction)
- Correction of deep bite
- Selected class II malocclusions
- Rapid adult orthodontics
- Rapid intrusion/extrusion of teeth
- Simultaneous correction of osseous and mucogingival defects
- Prevention of mucogingival defects that may occur during or after orthodontic treatment
- Multidisciplinary comprehensive treatments (incorporating generalized or localized Piezocision)

Contraindications

- Active periodontal disease
- Ankylosed teeth
- Systemic conditions affecting bone metabolism
- Medications affecting bone metabolism
- Noncompliant patient

Description of the Technique

A week after orthodontic appliances are placed, the patient is seen by the periodontist for piezocision surgery. Prior to the surgical appointment, the orthodontist and surgeon have discussed the case in depth, with the orthodontist telling the surgeon which teeth, or group of teeth, need to move and where. A preoperative CT scan is ideal as it will tell the team which teeth need bone grafting as well as give the surgeon information about the location of vital anatomical or critical dental structures (i.e. root form and proximity). This planning will lead to the making of the surgical flow chart (fig. 1) to be used as the blueprint for the surgical procedure. This sheet is carried to the operating room and used as a guide during the surgery.

Piezocision Surgery
The patient is requested to rinse with chlorhexidine gluconate 0.12% for 1 min before being given local anesthesia (fig. 2). Once anesthesia has set, with the help of a scalpel with a blade No. 15 interproximal buccal incisions are made in the attached gingiva or alveolar mucosa (this is dependent on the anatomy of the region and the amount of keratinized tissue present). The incisions are small enough to accomodate the diameter of the BS 1 insert of the piezotome (Satelec, Acteongroupe, Merignac, France). These incisions are started 2–3 mm below the base of the interproximal papillae, keeping in mind that the soft tissues and the underlying periosteum need to be cut to create an opening that will allow for the insertion of the BS 1 insert (fig. 3). Once all the superficial soft tissue incisions are completed, the piezotome is used to create the bone injury that will start the RAP. This is done by inserting the head of the BS1 insert in the gingival openings and decorticate the alveolar bone (fig. 4). The depth of the cut is

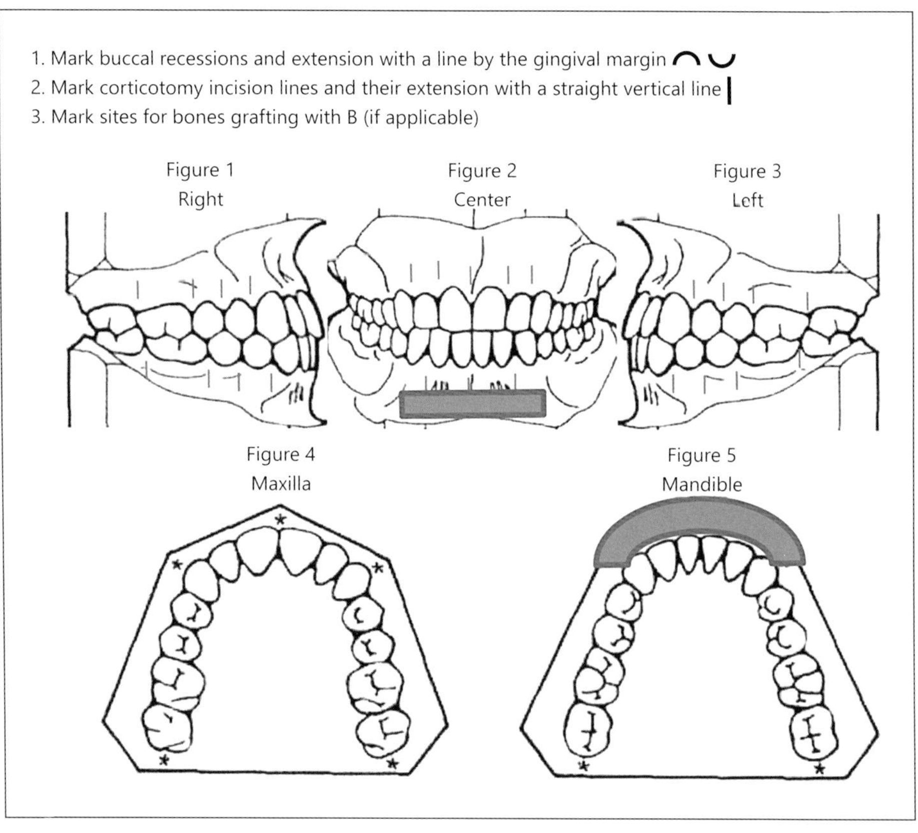

Fig. 1. Surgery Planning Chart (the interproximal Piezocision sites are marked by short vertical lines, and the areas needing bone grafting and shown in grey shading).

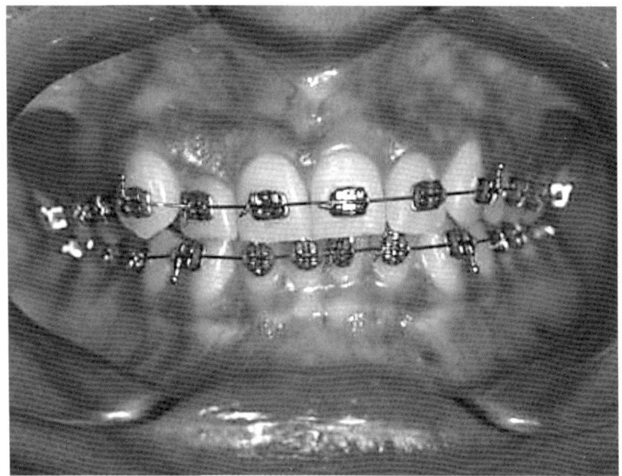

Fig. 2. 28-year-old patient presenting with a blocked out canine and a midline shift.

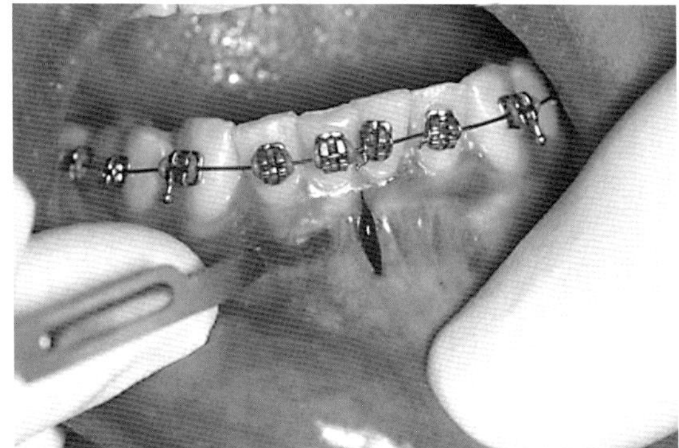

Fig. 3. Buccal and interproximal soft tissue incision with blade No. 15. The blade must cut through the periosteum in order to allow for bone decortication with the piezotome (Satelec, Acteongroup, Merignac, France).

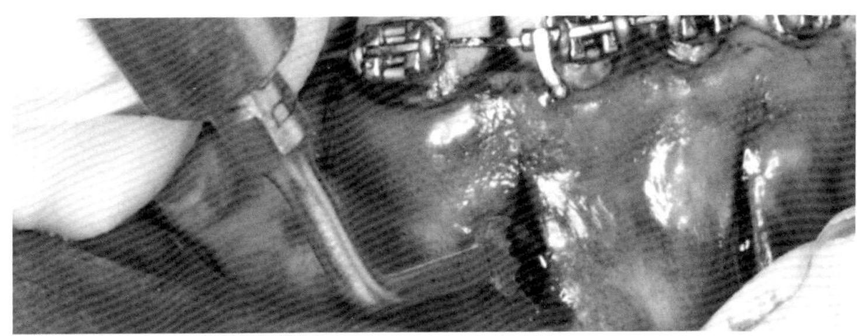

Fig. 4. The piezotome (Satelec, Acteongroup) with the BS1 insert is used to do the interproximal bony decortication that will start the RAP. Depth of cut: 3 mm.

3 mm. At this point, it is very important to pay attention to the direction of the bony cuts so as to not injure the surrounding roots. In the areas where bone augmentation is needed (this has been determined beforehand by the dental team after careful analysis of the preoperative CT scan), a subperiosteal tunneling procedure is performed (fig. 5). This is done by using a small periosteal elevator (24G, Hu Friedy, Chicago, Ill., USA) that is inserted in the vertical opening and below the periosteum. Care must be taken to create enough of a 'pouch' to accommodate the bone graft (fig. 6). By the same token, this tunneling procedure can be used to correct a pre-existing mucogingival defect (i.e. gingival recession) and a soft tissue graft from the palate is then inserted into the pouch instead of bone. Once the grafting procedure is completed, only the areas where tunneling was done need to be sutured with 5–0 chromic gut (fig. 7). The other areas (simple incisions with decortication) do not usually need suturing.

The postoperative regimen suggested is as follows:

- antibiotherapy (when bone grafting is done)
- nonsteroidal anti-inflammatory drugs to alleviate discomfort
- ice packs for the first 2 h after surgery
- rinses with chlorhexidine gluconate 0.12%.

Follow-Up Visits

There is a 1-week follow-up visit by the surgeon to assess proper healing. As of the second week after surgery, it is the orthodontist who will need to see the patient every 2 weeks for the next 4–6

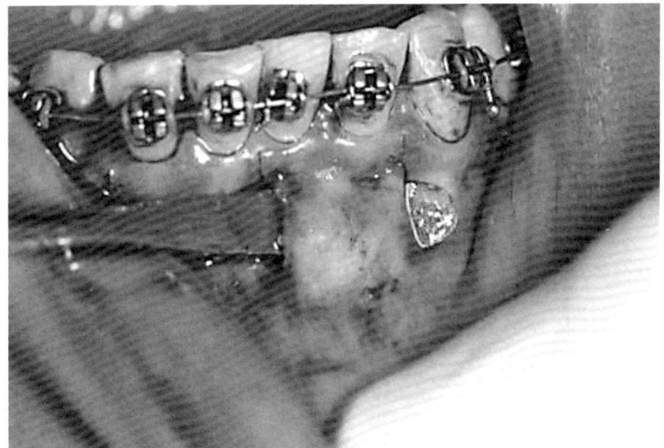

Fig. 5. Tunneling procedure using the periosteal elevator to create space for the bone graft that will also take place in that region.

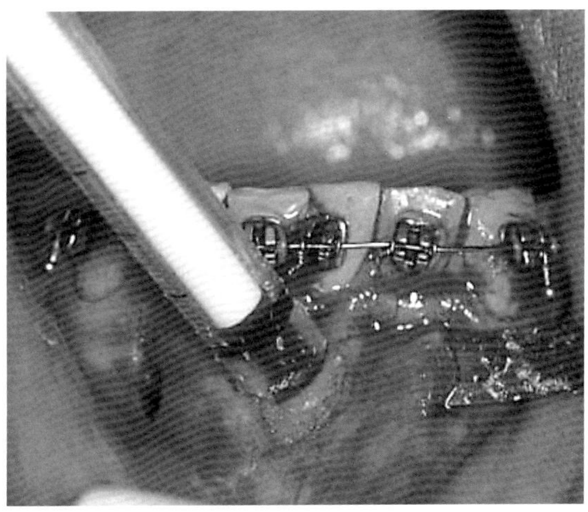

Fig. 6. A bone allograft (Regenafil, Exactech, Gainsville, Fla., USA) is being syringed into the prepared tunnel. This will augment the bone volume buccally and allow for anterior tooth movement at minimal risk for recessions.

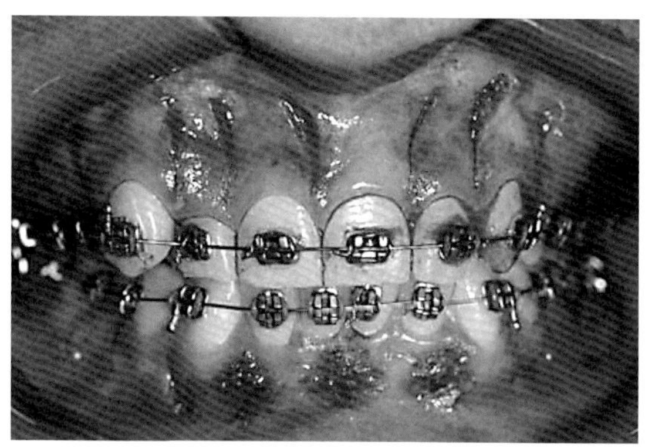

Fig. 7. The procedure is completed. The maxillary incisions should have been 50% smaller and not that high in the oral mucosa (as this will result in scarring). The lower anterior area that has been tunneled and grafted requires suturing. Here a few drops of cyanoacrylate glue have been added on top of the sutures.

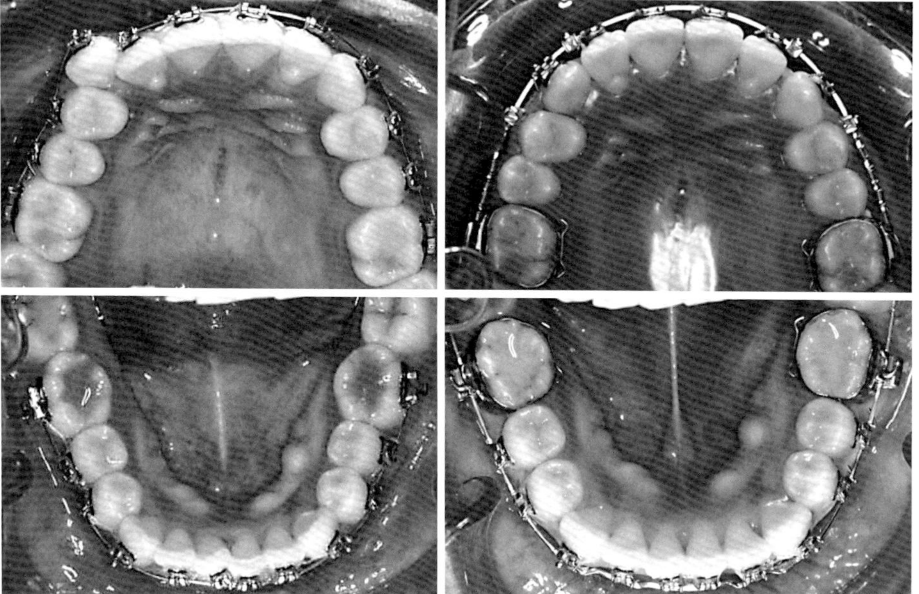

Fig. 8. Occlusal views before and 3.5 months after Piezocision. Notice that the upper right canine is on the arch and crowding has resolved (orthodontist: Dr. J.D. Sebaoun).

months. This is critical as we need to maximize tooth movement during this period of time. The RAP that follows bone decortication consists of two successive phases (catabolic and anabolic), and it is important to judiciously use the time during which the bone is demineralized (catabolic phase) in order to achieve the 'greater bulk' of tooth movement. This phase is estimated to take place 2 weeks after surgery and continue for up to 6 months thereafter; hence, the need to see the patient very frequently to maximize the use of this window of opportunity that will subsequently lead to early completion of treatment (fig. 8, 9). Unlike conventional orthodontics, and during the course of treatment, a sharp increase in tooth mobility is observed. This is the result of the transient osteopenia that occurs during the catabolic phase. It is a normal occurrence and should not

Dibart

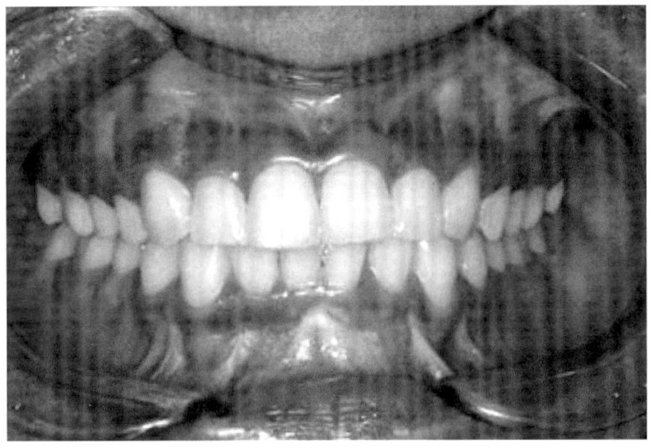

Fig. 9. Eight months after Piezocision the treatment is completed (orthodontist: Dr. J.D. Sebaoun).

trigger panic! It is to be expected and is temporary. This osteopenic effect is enhanced and prolonged, in time, by the orthodontic forces that are used during the treatment. These forces maintain mechanical stimulation of the alveolar bone; if these forces were not applied the demineralization phase will be shorter and less profound (data not shown).

Generalized versus Localized Piezocision

It is of paramount importance for the treatment planning team to understand that the surgically induced bone turnover is restricted to the surgical sites. This is important as bony incisions should only take place around teeth or group of teeth that will be moved. Piezocision can therefore be used for the whole mouth during conventional orthodontic treatment, the cuts being simultaneously performed at the maxilla and the mandible from second molar to second molar (see case illustrated here) or for segments of the dentition to achieve specific localized results (intrusion, extrusion, distalization of teeth, etc.). In this latter case, it is the judicious alteration and use of the relative anchorage value of teeth that will allow for successful outcome, as the relative anchorage value of teeth away from the surgical site remains high, and anchorage value of teeth close to the surgical site remains low.

Sequential Piezocision

In some cases, Piezocision can be used twice in the course of a single treatment, usually toward the end of the orthodontic treatment, once the RAP effect has long subsided and the orthodontist needs a 'booster' to finish the case. This is done in some areas of the dentition where specific and localized corrections are required (sequential Piezocision).

Conclusions

Piezocision is an innovative, minimally invasive surgical procedure that allows rapid orthodontic tooth movement without the down side of the extensive and traumatic classical surgical approach. Piezocision proves to be efficient from the patients and clinician's stand point and offers advantages that should lead to greater acceptance in the dental and patient communities.

References

1 Wilcko MT, Wilcko WM, Marquez MG, Ferguson DJ: The contribution of periodontics to orthodontic therapy; in Dibart S (ed): Practical Advanced Periodontal Surgery. Oxford, Wiley-Blackwell Publishing, 2007.

2 Wilcko WM, Wilcko T, Bouquot JE, Ferguson DJ: Rapid orthodontics with alveolar reshaping: two case reports of decrowding. Int J Periodontics Restorative Dent 2001;21:9–19.

3 Wilcko WM, Ferguson DJ, Bouguot JE, Wilcko MT: Rapid orthodontic decrowding with alveolar augmentation: case report. World J Orthodont 2003;4: 197–205.

4 Frost HA: The regional acceleratory phenomena: a review. Henry Ford Hosp Med J 1983;31:3–9.
5 Frost HM: The biology of fracture healing. An overview for clinicians. Part I. Clin Orthop Relat Res 1989;248:283–293.
6 Frost HM: The biology of fracture healing. An overview for clinicians. Part II. Clin Orthop Relat Res 1989;248:294–309.
7 Vercellotti T Podesta A: Orthodontic microsurgery: a new surgically guided technique for dental movement. Int J Periodontics Restorative Dent 2007;27:325–331.
8 Park YG, Kang SG, Kin SJ: Accelerated tooth movement by corticision as an osseous orthodontic paradigm. Kinki Tokai Kyosei Shika Gakkai Gakujyutsu Taikai, Sokai 2006;28:6.
9 Kim SJ, Park YG, Kang SG: Effects of corticision on paradental remodeling in orthodontic tooth movement. Angle Ortho 2009;79:284–291.
10 Dibart S, Sebaoun JD, Surmenian J: Piezocision: a minimally invasive, periodontally accelerated orthodontic tooth movement procedure. Compend Contin Educ Dent 2009;30:342–344, 346, 348–350.
11 Dibart S, Surmenian J, Sebaoun JD, Montesani L: Rapid treatment of class II malocclusion with Piezocision: two case reports. Int J Perio Restorative Dent 2010;30:487–493.
12 Keser EI, Dibart S: Piezocision-assisted Invisalign treatment. Compend Contin Educ Dent 2011;32:46–48, 50–51.

Serge Dibart, DMD
Department of Periodontology and Oral Biology
Boston University Henry M. Goldman School of Dental Medicine
100 East Newton Street, Boston, MA 02118 (USA)
E-Mail sdibart@bu.edu

Kantarci A, Will L, Yen S (eds): Tooth Movement. Front Oral Biol. Basel, Karger, 2016, vol 18, pp 109–117
DOI: 10.1159/000351904

Corticision: A Flapless Procedure to Accelerate Tooth Movement

Young Guk Park

Kyung Hee University School of Dentistry, Seoul, Korea

Abstract

Orthodontic tooth movement results from applied forces to the teeth evoking cellular responses in the teeth and their surrounding tissues, including the periodontal ligament, alveolar bone and gingiva. It is advantageous for the orthodontist to be well informed of the detailed process of the biological events that unfold during tooth movement, since some of these details may differ from one person to another due to biological differences such as periodontal metabolism or alveolar bone density. This led us to emphasize that orthodontics is a field of endeavor where the integration of mechanics and biology is materialized, and to affirm the fact that tooth movement is conducted in individual human beings, each composed of a unique and intricate physiological system. Biological variations may be the foundation of the differences that are frequently observed in the outcomes of orthodontic treatment in particular with reference to treatment duration between patients with similar malocclusions and who were treated identically. A wide diversity of clinical trials has been carried out to control the tissue resistance to facilitate orthodontic tooth movement, which involves biomechanical, pharmaceutical, surgical, electrical regimens or tissue engineering technology. The term 'Corticision' is a neologism which indicates 'cortical bone incision'. It is a minimally invasive periodontal procedure without flap elevation, thus accelerating tooth movement with an enhanced turnover rate of the surrounding structures. This chapter introduces the technical procedure, and the biological background of how such a minor surgical procedure can receive the accelerated tooth movement with impunity and thereby shorten the duration of treatment.
© 2016 S. Karger AG, Basel

Orthodontic tooth movement results by applying mechanical forces applied on the teeth which evoke cellular responses in the teeth and their surrounding tissues, including the periodontal ligament, alveolar bone and gingiva. The biological cascades along with the conventional protocols of biomechanics yield tooth movement by approximately 1 mm per month which may require about 2–3 years of treatment. Most orthodontic patients prefer to wear orthodontic braces for as short a period as possible. A great variety of clinical trials have put a vast amount of effort into reducing this period by 30–50%. Previous reports have demonstrated that such a target is attainable when orthodontic forces are applied together with subjecting the periodontal tissues to surgical and/or tissue engineering procedures; nonetheless, these procedures involve relatively complicated surgical regimens of full-thickness flap and extensive alveolar bone decortication.

Recently, a wide diversity of clinical trials to accelerate tooth movement with a minimally invasive periodontal-orthodontic procedure without flap elevation has been suggested. All the trials have focused on making the milieu clinically expedient, and rendering the treatment duration shorter and less prone to complications. The aim of this chapter is to introduce the minimally invasive procedure, which has been named 'Corticision' by the author, to accelerate periodontal turnover rate without tissue damage during orthodontic treatment, and to demonstrate the technical procedure and risk management when performing the procedure in actual patients to enhance the rate of bony and periodontal response, thereby shortening the duration of treatment.

Development of the Concept

The surgically assisted orthodontics for facilitating orthodontic tooth movement were adopted by Cohn-Stock in 1921, removing the palatal bone on the maxillary teeth to expedite retraction of the anterior teeth. A generative description, published by Köle [1] in 1959, summarizes a decortication of the alveolar process to promote tooth movement. Adding some conspicuous rectification, this procedure has become the fundamental technique adopted today by those who advocate the merger of orthodontic treatment and periodontal surgery. In 1972, Bell and Levy [2] studied the corticotomy techniques luxating the tooth-bearing bone segments with a chisel in *Macaca mulatta*, and denoted a destructive effect on the maxillary incisors. They stated a compromised circulation in the intraosseous and intrapulpal structures; however, they did not substantiate clinically remarkable damage. On the contrary, Wilcko et al. [3] accentuated that there was no luxation of the bone, since the luxation of the tooth-bearing bone segment signifies an irrational mechanical justification and does not fit the purpose of decortication which aims to alter the bone physiology. Düker [4] repeated Köle's experiment in dogs in exactly the same way and reported the movement of an incisor segment to be 4 mm in 8–20 days without periodontal breakdown or loss of vitality of the pulp.

Merrill and Pedersen [5] scrutinized the procedure for immediate repositioning of dental-osseous elements, laying stress on the safety of the osteotomy and immediate repositioning of the dentoalveolar complex. They reported some unspecified complications which, they stated, did not suffice to denounce the procedure. The authors suggested accomplishment of the interdental osteotomies first on the buccal aspect and then on the lingual side of the alveolus which was expected to provide collateral circulation with a vascular anastomosis, and this idea was considered to be a meaningful alternative.

In 1978, Generson et al. [6] reported treatment of the anterior open bite by the decortication procedure where the bony cut was performed though the cortical layer to preserve the viability of bone segments by leaving the marrow intact.

Much later in 1985, Mostafa et al. [7] described a surgical orthodontic approach to treat over-erupted maxillary molars, where the decortication procedure was localized to the alveolus of a single tooth, the extruded molar. This was citable in the context of the procedure to work for a single tooth. Two years later, in 1987, Goldson and Reck [8] reported surgical-orthodontic treatment of malpositioned cuspids. The authors presented a segmental mucoperiosteal flap to separate the entire dentoalveolar segment through the buccal cortex and medullary bone. A collateral blood supply from the adjacent mucoperiosteum was sufficient to maintain the viability of the segment.

No remarkable development after Köle's work was suggested until Suya [9] introduced 'corticotomy-facilitated orthodontics'. He exclusively counted on the effects of linear interproximal decortication without connecting the buccal and lingual cuts in about 300 patients. This modification had essentially been designated the gold standard for decortication procedures, and, as Köle [1] and Suya [9] noted, it accelerated the rate of tooth movement.

Early in the present century, Thomas and William Wilcko [10, 11] of Erie, Pennsylvania, marked a new era at the beginning of unprecedented contributions. Based on the Köle and Suya technique, they added the resorbable augmentation mixture as a bone graft to the procedure with the objective of attracting cells to the area where the new bone formation was needed, ensuring a sound periodontal support. The hypotheses of Frost [12] were employed to explain the accelerated periodontal response around the orthodontically treated teeth. Ferguson et al. [13] carried out retrospective studies on the clinical efficacy and safety of the Wilcko-rectified technique, which was named 'Accelerated Osteogenic Orthodontics™' and is also known as 'Periodontally Accelerated Osteogenic Orthodontics™'. It is important to note that placement of the graft mixture is a compulsory measure to decortication procedures, where the structural integrity of the supporting periodontium is preserved and strengthened. Simple decortication, i.e. almost any kind of intentional injury, to hard or soft tissue, is sufficient to elicit a regional acceleratory phenomenon (RAP) commensurate with the degree of trauma.

Germec et al. [14] reported a modified corticotomy, where they represented a conservative corticotomy technique to facilitate the rate of tooth movement during lower incisor retraction. After extraction of the four first premolars, corticotomy was performed without lingual cuts. This modification dramatically reduced treatment duration without any detrimental effects on the periodontium and teeth. The main advantage of this technique is reduced postoperative morbidity, by eliminating lingual cuts and flap. This is a pertinent modification, because the RAP of Frost [12] is sufficiently brought out for this type of tooth movement. The use of minimal intervention to achieve a given objective suggests a keen knowledge of the RAP physiology and respect for a discrete surgical technique. Germec's technique focused on the importance of the psychosocial aspect critical for patient compliance by reducing the operation time and minimizing patient discomfort.

The concept of 'bony-block' tooth movement was dismissed after the Loma Linda studies. Ferguson et al. [13] characterized the regional acceleratory phenomenon as an increased anabolic modeling of the alveolus adjacent to the selective alveolar decortication area in the study using a rat model. The amplification of anabolic activity in the rat appeared to increase by 150% at 3 weeks. This increase represented about a 2- to 3-fold greater anabolic modeling activity in the spongious bone compared to a same-animal contralateral control. Sebaoun et al. [15] reported a 200% rise in spongious catabolic activity and a 400% increase in osteoblastic activity was noted at 3 weeks in the rat model. It was concluded that this effect demonstrates the mechanism of rapid tooth movement. This is based on a reasonable assumption that under a fixed orthodontic force teeth move faster through bone undergoing surgical healing because either decreased bone density yields less tissue resistance, or increased local metabolism mediates enhanced periodontal turnover along with orthodontic tooth movement.

Corticision

The term, corticotomy, has been appearing a lot in the previous clinical literature with its inconsistent use for various cases of clinical and research protocols. It reflects the semantic obscurity historically. The term surgically assisted orthodontics is meant to encompass all

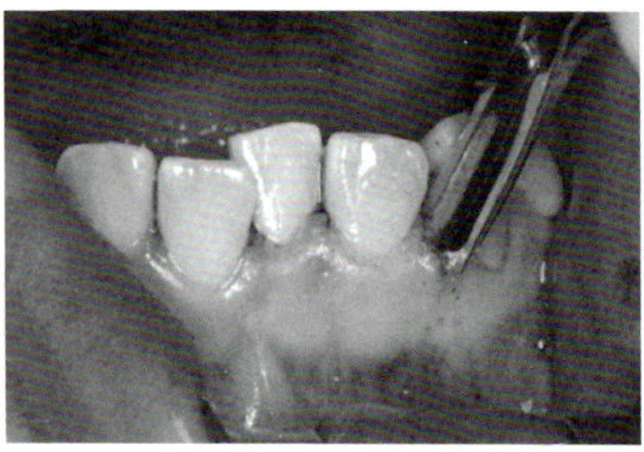

Fig. 1. The Corticision. The interradicular cortical bone is cut transmucosally without flap elevation.

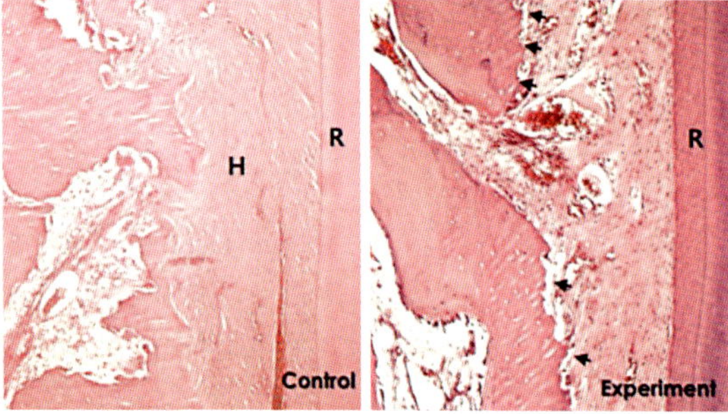

Fig. 2. Seven days after the Corticision in a cat. The compressed PDL in the experimental (Corticision) group manifested less hyalinized tissue and more viable cells than the control group, resulting in direct bone resorption. H = Hyalinization; R = root. HE. ×100. Cited from the author's own publication: Angle Orthod 2009;79:287.

dentoalveolar surgical procedures of periodontal tissues around orthodontic treatment. One of the surgically assisted orthodontics is selective alveolar decortication which is the procedure designed to alter bone physiology and accelerate the rate of tooth movement. The term corticotomy is reserved for those periodontal surgeries that incise deep into the medullary bone with a chisel or osteotomy, whether luxation is included or not.

The purpose of selective alveolar decortication is to manipulate the physiology by initiating a healing state known as RAP, an osteopenic state of accelerated bone metabolism maintained by the trauma of tooth movement and enhanced by the introduction of intentional surgical damage. Thus, the primary purpose of the surgical manipulation is not attempting to reassemble or rearrange the target alveolar parts in a new spatial position. Accordingly, the concept that selective alveolar decortication produces movement of 'bony block or dentoalveolar segment in space' is no longer accepted in our clinical and research avenue. The evidence that the alteration of the bony milieu around teeth is by virtue of altered physiology is submitted by the relevant studies [16–18]. The review of the history of surgical attempts to facilitate orthodontic treatment is befitting when it comes to defining the principal objectives of stability and efficient tooth movement.

In spite of all the favorable changes in bone physiology after the surgically assisted orthodontics, all these procedures accompany full-thickness flap elevation. The mucoperiosteal flap elevation per se give rise to widening of the periodontal ligament space, increased tooth mobility and bone dehiscence, as mentioned by Yaffe et al. [19]. The authors have introduced a procedure, named 'Corticision', wherein a reinforced scalpel is used as a thin chisel to separate the interproximal cortices transmucosally, without a flap reflection, as depicted in figure 1. The Corticision was conceived by the suggestion that the very drawback along with flap surgery in the conventional procedures may be overcome by cutting the interradicular cortical bone without periodontal surgery for full-thickness flap elevation. Transmucosal manipulation of the alveolar bone minimizes morbidity and is found to recruit the regional acceleratory phenomenon.

The 'Corticision' also submits that the alteration of the bony milieu around teeth is attributable to altered physiology based on the author's own study [20, 21]. Figure 2 depicts that the Corticision evokes catabolic remodeling in the compression side of tooth movement accompanied by direct bone resorption, less hyalinization, and expeditious disappearance of the hyalinized molds in cats which signifies instant elimination of frontal bone matrix. The Corticision promotes the anabolic remodeling activity, particularly at the

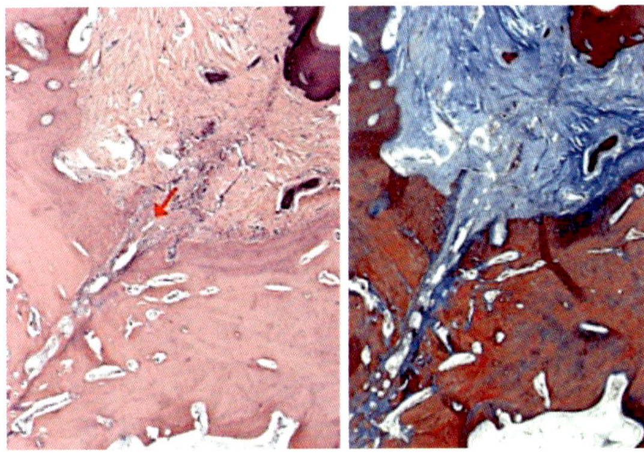

Fig. 3. 21 days after the Corticision in a cat. Healing of Corticision site in the tension side of the canine. Surgical gap (arrow) by the Corticision was almost filled with new bone. Overlying soft tissue was recovered. HE and Trichrome. ×40. Cited from the author's own publication: Angle Orthod 2009;79:289.

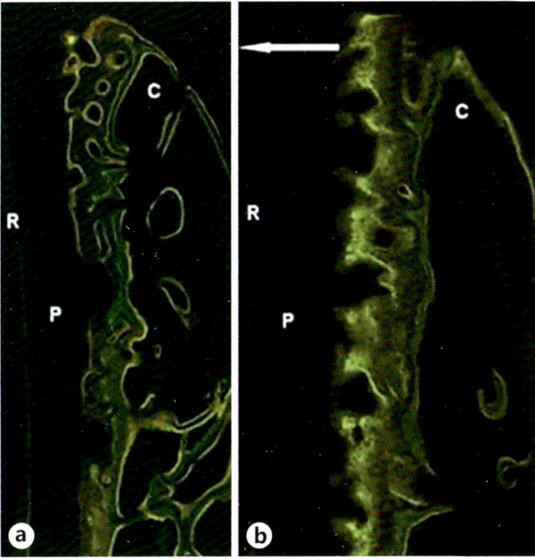

Fig. 4. Microphotographs of fluorescence in tension side at 28 days after the Corticision in cat. **a** Control group. **b** Corticision group. More new bone was formed in the Corticision group than in the control. R = Root; P = periodontal ligament; C = cementum. Cited from the author's own publication: Angle Orthod 2009;79:290.

tension side in cats, as illustrated in figure 3. The surgical gap produced by the Corticision is filled with newly formed woven bone which will be transformed into mature lamellar bone. Apposition of newly mineralized bone matrix in the tension side at 28 days after the Corticision in a cat model is well presented in figure 4. The mean apposition area of the mineralized matrix appears 3-fold more than in a normal orthodontic group.

Technical Procedure

The armamentarium involves a reinforced scalpel (No. 15T, Paragon, Sheffield, UK) and an ordinary scalpel holder as well as a surgical mallet, as shown in figure 5. Panoramic X-rays or serial periapical radiograms are mandatory to check the available interradicular room for carrying out the procedure. A preoperative antiseptic mouth rinse is recommended for prevention of potential infection. After infiltration anesthesia, position the scalpel on the interradicular attached gingiva at an inclination of 45–60° to the long axis of the tooth to be moved (fig. 6), and

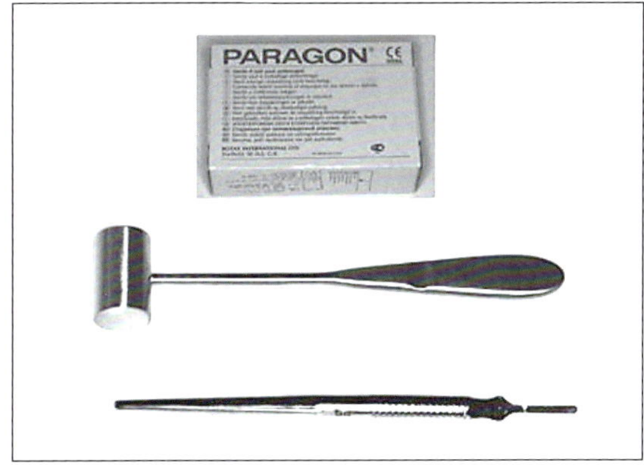

Fig. 5. Armamentarium for the Corticision.

insert it gradually into the bone marrow by tapping the scalpel holder with the surgical mallet, passing through the overlying gingiva and cortical bone, and into the cancellous bone. The vertical cut leaves 5 mm of the papillary gingiva to avoid bone loss of the alveolar crest and

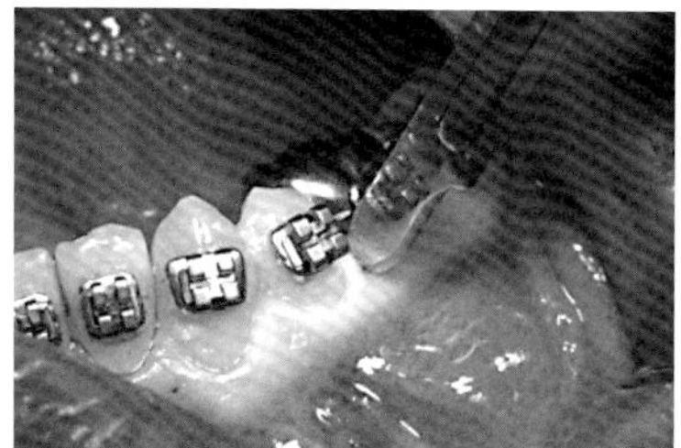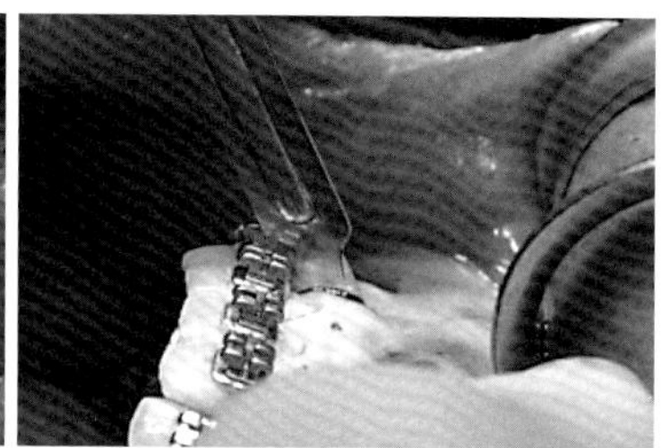

Fig. 6. Place the blade at a right angle to the gingival surface, then turn obliquely at 45–60° down towards the apex, which helps the longer cut into the medullary bone with minimal soft tissue (gingival) injury.

consequent development of the 'black triangle' and damage of the adjacent dental root (fig. 7). The depth of alveolar penetration with the scalpel is about 10 mm for the sake of beneficial cancellous bone osteotomy, which is expected to generate new blood vessels and enhance trabecular bone remodeling. Since the length of the vertical cut in the interradicular attached gingiva is not necessarily the entire root length, 2/3 of the root length is sufficient to evoke rapid tooth movement. After the Corticision receives its sufficient vertical cut, pull out the scalpel with a gentle swing motion. Figure 8 describes that there is no conspicuous bleeding or troubled soft tissue left, thereby not requiring any postoperative dressing such as suture or periodontal pack. As the final step, mild irrigation with normal saline for a couple of minutes is required until the cessation of bleeding or oozing. When the 'Corticision' is planned at the beginning of the treatment, the procedure is preferred to be accomplished immediately after bonding in order to avoid a moistened enamel surface. Upon finishing, place the initial archwire with comfort.

The effect of tooth movement in the context of velocity with the Corticision is postulated to be dose dependent as in any other procedures for selective alveolar decortication by the study of Hazenberg et al. [17]. The bigger intensive cortical bone cut along with the entire length of the dental root will bring considerable periodontal turnover, a higher likelihood of soft tissue injury and a potential risk of postoperative complications such as infection that vitality loss of the adjacent

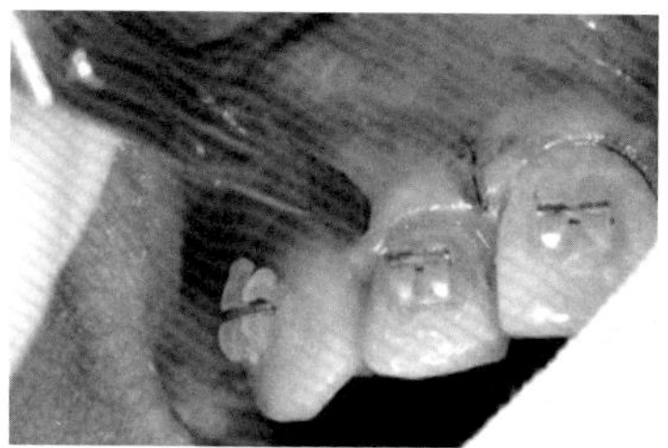

Fig. 7. The scalpel penetrates about 10 mm in depth to obtain a cortical bone as well as a cancellous bone cut. The Corticision begins 5 mm downwards to the papillary gingiva to keep the papillary gingiva intact.

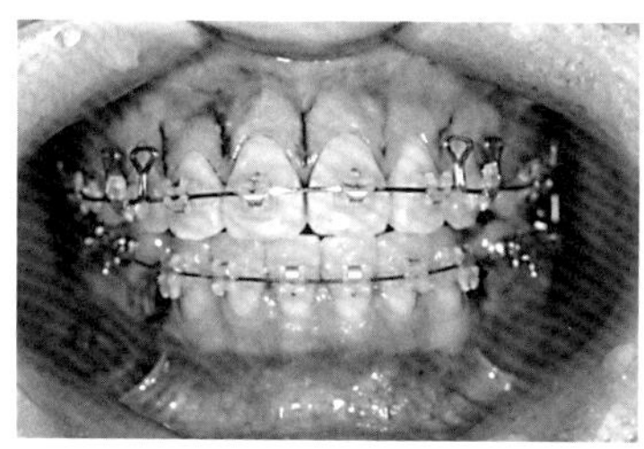

Fig. 8. Immediately after the Corticision. Note there is no conspicuous postoperative bleeding.

tooth may bring. Henceforth, the intentional damage is recommended to be at the break-even point level, which dictates the length of the vertical cut to be 2/3 of the root length. Figure 9 represents the intraoral view of crowding relieved with the Corticision in a fairly short period of time. Figure 10 illustrates how the Corticison works in the case of bicuspid extraction.

The biomechanics after the Corticision do not necessarily signify an exaggerated force

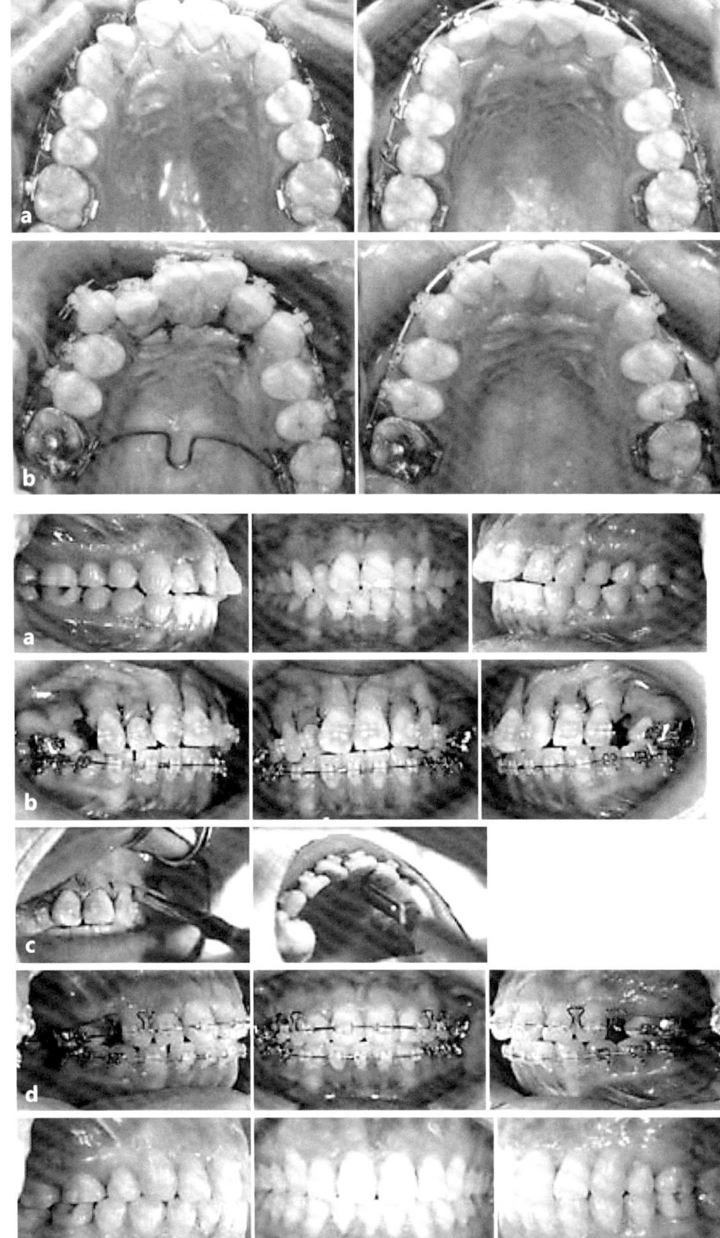

Fig. 9. Intraoral photos before and after the Corticision. Mild crowding was completely relieved in 3 weeks (**a**), while moderate crowding took 9 weeks for complete alleviation (**b**).

Fig. 10. Intraoral photos of a case, 21-year-old female, with crowding and anterior protrusion before (**a**), at bonding and upper bicuspid extraction (**b**), at Corticision (**c**), 3 months after treatment (**d**) and at debonding 10 months after treatment (**e**). The Corticision was performed on the upper arch at the beginning of treatment.

level. The ordinary mechanical system for each orthodontist's preference yields an identical treatment outcome except for the short time period. The overall effect from the Corticision reaches at its peak at 2 months and drops at 3 months when the procedure is carried out. During the 3 months of this effective period, the patients are advised to visit every other week in order to keep the Corticision gap by the woven bone open, otherwise the woven bone transforms

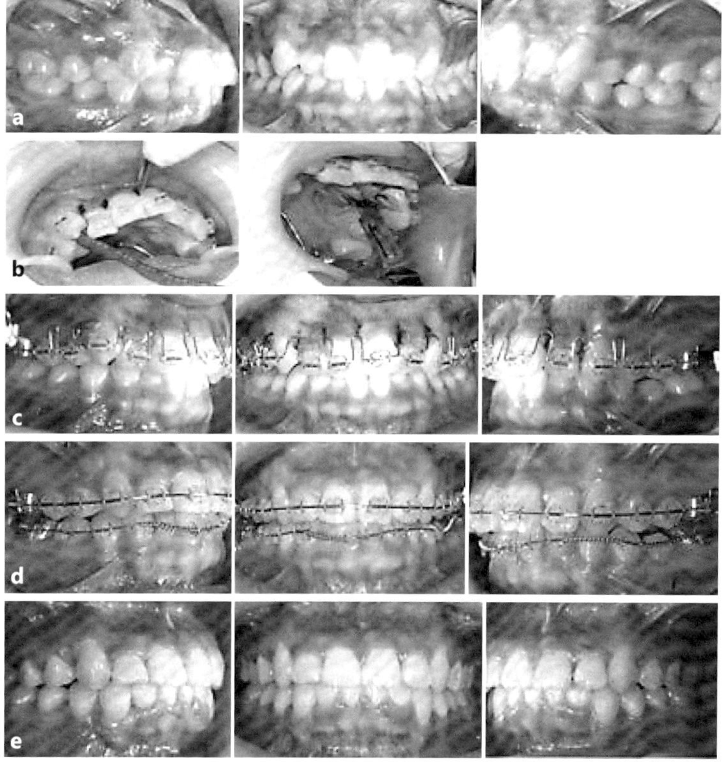

Fig. 11. Intraoral photos of a case with crowding, 21-year-old female, before (**a**), on the day (**c**) and 2 months after the Corticision (**d**), and debonding at 10 months after treatment (**e**). The Corticision (**b**) was performed on the upper arch at the beginning of treatment.

into mature lamellar bone at 3 weeks after gap formation, leading to a sharp decline of the effects.

Risk Management

The Corticision is classified as the high risk level of infection according to the 'Consensus document on the use of antibiotic prophylaxis in dental surgery and procedure' by the Center for Disease Control and Prevention (US) in 2006. This denotes that the prescription of prophylactic, broad-spectrum antibiotics such as amoxicillin with the appropriate analgesics is mandatory. Special consideration in choice of pain killer is imperative since nonsteroidal anti-inflammatory drugs (NSAIDs) are consequently known to inhibit bone resorption and retard tooth move-

ment, whereas acetaminophen has been proven to not affect the rate of tooth movement. The best choice of drug to control postoperative pain/discomfort is Tylenol™. There is hardly an opportunity to observe any scarring in the oral mucosa or to follow any detrimental sequelae due to fibrous scar banding.

Conclusion

Figure 11 depicts a 21-year-old female patient who has received the Corticision and an ordinary biomechanical regimen, finishing her treatment within 10 months. The diminution of treatment duration is attributable to the RAP which stimulates periodontal turnover and a consequently well-disposed environment for tooth movement. Previous studies embodied the consensus that intentional injury to the periodontium leads to lower bone density by transient osteopenia increasing bone volume and thus providing a favorable microenvironment for accelerated tooth movement. The fact that the RAP dominantly takes place at the cortical bone enabled the conception of Corticision – minimally invasive, intentional surgical injury without flap elevation while sufficient to elicit the necessary tissue response.

Any measurement which evokes cellular recruitment in the alveolar bone may accelerate tooth movement. Such a measure is best adopted in clinical practice if the intervention is minimal with less discomfort and there are no adverse effects on the patients. Corticision is believed to meet this imperative biological prerequisite exactly.

Acknowledgement

The author would like to extend his heartfelt gratitude to his forever mentor, Dr. Ze'ev Davidovitch, a clinical Professor at Case Western Reserve University, for his unsparing teachings and inspiration.

References

1 Köle H: Surgical operations of the alveolar ridge to correct occlusal abnormalities. Oral Surg Oral Med Oral Pathol 1959;12:515–529.

2 Bell WH, Levy BM: Revascularization and bone healing after maxillary corticotomies. J Oral Surg 1972;30:640–648.

3 Wilcko WM, Wilcko MT, Bouquot JE, Ferguson DJ: Accelerated orthodontics with alveolar reshaping. J Ortho Pract 2000;10:63–70.

4 Düker J: Experimental animal research into segmental alveolar movement after corticotomy. J Maxillofac Surg 1975;3:81–84.

5 Merrill RG, Pedersen GW: Interdental osteotomy for immediate repositioning of dental-osseous elements. J Oral Surg 1976;34:118–125.

6 Generson RM, Porter JM, Zell A, Stratigos GT: Combined surgical and orthodontic management of anterior open bite using corticotomy. J Oral Surg 1978;36:216–219.

7 Mostafa YA, Tawfik KM, El-Mangoury NH: Surgical-orthodontic treatment for overerupted maxillary molars. J Clin Orthod 1985;19:350–351.

8 Goldson L, Reck VJ: Surgical-orthodontic treatment of malpositioned cuspids. J Clin Orthod 1987;21:847–851.

9 Suya H: Corticotomy in orthodontics; in Hosl E, Baldauf A (eds): Mechanical and Biological Basics in Orthodontic Therapy. Heidelberg, Huthig Buch Verlag, Germany, 1991, pp 207–226.

10 Wilcko WM, Wilcko MT, Bouquot JE, Ferguson DJ: Accelerated orthodontics with alveolar reshaping. J Ortho Pract 2000;10:63–70.

11 Wilcko WM, Wilcko T, Bouquot JE, Ferguson DJ; Rapid orthodontics with alveolar reshaping: two case reports of decrowding. Int J Periodontics Restorative Dent 2001;21:9–19.

12 Frost HM: The regional acceleratory phenomenon: a review. Henry Ford Hosp Med J 1983;31:3–9.

13 Ferguson DJ, Sebaoun J-D, Turner JW, Kantarci A, Carvalho RS, Van Dyke TE: Anabolic Modeling of Trabecular Bone following Selective Alveolar Decortication. Orlando, ADEA/AADR/CADR, 2006, paper 0768.

14 Germec D, Giray B, Kocadereli I, Enacar A: lower incisor retraction with a modified corticotomy. Angle Orthod 2006;76:880–888.

15 Sebaoun JD, Kantarci A, Turner JW, Carvalho RS, Van Dyke TE, Ferguson DJ: Modeling of trabecular bone lamina dura following selective alveolar decortication in rats. J Periodontol 2008;79:1679–1688.

16 Lee W, Karapetyan G, Moats R, Yamashita DD, Moon HB, Ferguson DJ, Yen S: Corticotomy-/osteotomy-assisted tooth movement microCTs differ. J Dent Res 2008;87:861–867.

17 Hazenberg JG, Freeley M, Foran E, Lee TC, Taylor D: Microdamage: cell transducing mechanism based on ruptured osteocyte processes. J Biomech 2006;39:209.

18 Murphy KG, Wilcko MT, Wilcko WM, Ferguson DJ: Periodontal accelerated osteogenic orthodontics: a description of the surgical technique. J Oral Maxillofac Surg 2009;67:2160–2166.

19 Yaffe A, Fine N, Binderman I: Regional accelerated phenomenon in the mandible following mucoperiosteal flap surgery. J Periodontol 1994;65:79–83.

20 Kim SJ, Park YG, Kang SG: Effects of Corticision on paradental remodeling in orthodontic tooth movement. Angle Orthod 2009;79:284–291.

21 Kim SJ, Moon SU, Kang SG, Park YG: Effects of low level laser therapy after Corticision on tooth movement and paradental remodeling. Lasers Surg Med 2009;41:524–533.

Prof. Young Guk Park
Department of Orthodontics, Kyung Hee University School of Dentistry
Hoeki Dong 1
Seoul 130-701 (Korea)
E-Mail ygpark@khu.ac.kr

Kantarci A, Will L, Yen S (eds): Tooth Movement. Front Oral Biol. Basel, Karger, 2016, vol 18, pp 118–123
DOI: 10.1159/000351906

Photobiomodulation and Lasers

Susanne Chiari

Department of Orthodontics, Bernhard Gottlieb University Clinic of Dentistry, Medical University of Vienna, Vienna, Austria

Abstract

Photobiomodulation is discussed to be a noninvasive method to accelerate orthodontic tooth movement. The stimulatory effect of low-level laser therapy is well known and includes enhancement in tissue growth and tissue regeneration, resolvement of inflammation and pain. In recent research projects, the effect of laser therapy was tested regarding the stimulatory effect on bone remodeling with the potential to influence the tooth movement rate. The results are divers. The effect of laser regarding the reduction of the postadjustment pain could be proved, but not all authors describe the acceleration of tooth movement. Depending on the protocol, low-level laser therapy with low dosage increases the amount of tooth movement while high dosage seems to result in inhibitory effects. In conclusion, future studies are neces sary to find the right protocol delivering beneficial results regarding the influence on bone remodeling and tooth movement to implement this therapy in daily orthodontic routine.
© 2016 S. Karger AG, Basel

Accelerating tooth movement is of significant interest to orthodontists and especially to patients and has recently been the focus of different research studies. As described above in detail, there are different approaches to increase the rate of tooth movement and reduce orthodontic treatment time. Consequently, an improvement in patients' comfort, lower risk of root resorption and less risk of negative consequences due to the more complicated oral hygiene can be expected. On the one hand, there are nonsurgical methods using biochemical agents such as local injection of prostaglandins [1, 2], local injection of $1,25(OH)_2D_3$ [3, 4] or local injection of osteocalcin and alterations in alveolar calcium metabolism [5]. On the other hand, there are surgical techniques, which cause bone loss and reduce bone density with the aim to speed up tooth movement.

Another recent therapeutic approach to enhance the rate of tooth movement is the technique of photobiomodulation also known as phototherapy or laser therapy [6–8]. The exposure to low-level laser light is described to be a noninvasive method, which is painless and is not associated with any systemic effects. Furthermore, it is described to be simple to perform and not requiring expensive equipment [9].

In the following part, the stimulatory mechanism of the low-level laser therapy should be described as well as the effects on orthodontic therapy seen in animal studies and clinical trials should be embraced. Finally, the results of different research projects should be discussed and future perspectives of this method should be given.

Photobiomodulatory Effects

Low-level laser therapy is claimed to have beneficial biostimulatory effects such as enhanced tissue growth and tissue regeneration including soft tissue and bone regeneration, resolve inflammation and reduce pain. As bone remodeling places an important role during tooth movement in orthodontic therapy the stimulatory effect of laser therapy seems to have the potential to influence orthodontic treatment time [10]. However, the mechanism of the laser irradiation on bone remodeling has not been elucidated in detail and therefore was topic of recent research projects. Saito et al. [11] proved the stimulatory effect of laser treatment to bone regeneration in the mid-palatal suture during rapid maxillary expansion in rats. Furthermore, Ozawa et al. [10] looked at the effects of pulsed laser irradiation on bone formation at various stages of differentiating cells from rat fetal calvariae. They found out that there is a stimulating effect on bone formation included a cellular proliferation at an early stage, especially of nodule-forming cells of osteoblast lineage and an increased status of cellular differentiation resulting in a higher range of differentiated osteoblastic cells and therefore a higher rate of bone formation. When the same group [8] looked at the effect of bone acceleration after low-level laser irradiation during tooth movement in rats, they found an increased rate in tooth movement in the irradiation compared to the nonirradiation group accompanied by an acceleration of bone formation and resorption. In this study, an increase in the number of osteoclasts, cellular proliferation and mineralized bone formation showed an accelerating effect of laser therapy not only concerning the bone formation at the tension side but also the resorptive activity at the compression side of the moved tooth. Ninomiya et al. [12] pointed out that the biological effect of the laser light depends on the characteristics of the light source such as wavelength, output power and energy density and different laser systems are associated with different biostimulatory effects. The authors looked at the effect of a nanosecond pulsed laser light and found out that the bone volume in the femur of a rat could be increased by nanosecond pulsed laser light [13]. Furthermore, trabecular thickness, mineral apposition rate, bone mineral density and stress strain indices in the rat femur were accelerated. Concordant with the previously described study, it could be concluded that the effect was related to a higher osteoblast activity and a decrease in osteoclast number. Furthermore, Fujita et al. [7] examined the effect of laser irradiation on osteoclastogenesis. Especially, they looked at the expression of RANK, RANKL, and OPG during tooth movement accompanied by low-level laser irradiation. RANKL, a cytokine belonging to the tumor necrosis factor family is essential for the induction of osteoclastogenesis produced by osteoblasts and bone marrow cells. The signals are transduced by the specific receptor RANK, which is localized on the cell surface of osteoclast progenitors. OPG on the other hand, also produced by osteoblasts and bone marrow stromal cells, inhibits osteoclastogenesis by being involved in the binding of RANK with RANKL. The results of this study suggest that the acceleration of tooth movement under laser irradiation therapy may be affected by RANKL/RANK expression, whereas OPG-positive cells were not different among the irradiation and nonirradiation groups. Another important aspect in osteoclastogenesis was examined by Yamaguchi et al. [6] who found an increased rate of tooth movement together with an expression of MMP9, cathepsin K, and integrin subunits of $\alpha(v)\beta3$ expression. Beside the aspect of bone formation, maintenance of the periodontium seems to be an important aspect during tooth movement and, therefore, the balance between proliferation and differentiation of the extracellular matrix is important. In an in vivo study, Marquezan et al. [9] looked at the effect of two different low-level therapy protocols, one with daily irradiation and one with irradiation only during the early stages. While they did not find acceleration in tooth movement in any group they saw an increase in the number of osteoclasts after day 7 and an inhibition of the expression of immature collagen on the tension side. Furthermore, Habib et al. [14] who looked at the histological changes in the alveolar bone during tooth movement accompanied by irradiation therapy they found an increased number of osteoclasts on the pressure side of the irradiation group compared to nonirradiated animals as well as a significant increase in the osteoblast number on the tension side as well as higher amounts of collagen matrix on the pressure side. Kim et al. [15] investigated the effects of low-level laser light on the tissue turnover rate during tooth movement in rats and suggested that the connective tissue turnover could be facilitated with an increase expression of fibronectin and collagen type I due to the light application.

Photobiomodulation in Orthodontics

The photobiomodulative effect of low-level laser therapy has been of special interest in orthodontic therapy in recent years. On the one hand, orthodontic patients often feel pain and discomfort in response to the orthodontic forces delivered by the fixed appliances. On the other hand, the reduction of treatment time by accelerating orthodontic tooth movement is an important topic for reducing the discomfort of fixed appliances themselves and the risk of negative side effects of an elongated treatment, such as root resorption or consequences of a more difficult oral hygiene.

The postadjustment pain of orthodontic appliances is often the reason that patients avoid the orthodontic treatment itself [16, 17] or from preventing the patient from a sufficient plaque control. In a clinical study, Lim et al. [18] tested the efficiency of low-level laser treatment with three different treatment durations of 15, 30 and 60 s on controlling the postadjustment pain of orthodontic patients. The immediate pain relieve as well as the effect on the time course of pain intensity was tested over 5 days. The results showed a weak trend in lower pain scores and lower increases in pain intensity but the therapy was not able to provide immediate pain relief. Turhani et al. [19] tested the single application of low-level laser irradiation for 30 s per banded tooth and evaluated the pain perception after 6, 30 and 54 h. The prevalence of pain could be reduced after 6 and 30 h, but no significant difference was reported for the pain perception after 54 h. The effect of LLT on the pain intensity could not be evaluated in this study. In another clinical study, the effect of laser irradiation on the pain level was tested during canine retraction. In this study, the laser regime included an application at 0-, 3-, 7- and 14-day intervals. The results confirmed that in different treatment stages the pain level could be lowered on the side of laser application compared to the control side without irradiation therapy. Another study [20] tested the pain reducing effect of CO_2 laser applications in patients and found a reduction in pain from immediately after insertion of separators through day 4, but no difference on the non-irradiated control side could be registered thereafter. In a second study [21], the effect of CO_2 laser irradiation on the early responses to nociceptive stimuli during tooth movement was investigated and a significant reduction of the number of Fos-IR neurons 2 h after tooth movement in rats accompanied with CO_2 laser irradiation could be found. It could be concluded that irradiation therapy has the potential of reducing the early response to nociceptive stimuli during tooth movement without any negative side effect on the periodontal tissue.

To accelerate orthodontic tooth movement has become an important aim of recent research projects with the objective to reduce treatment time and have more compliant and satisfied patients without the risk of further complications due to elongated orthodontic treatment. There are only a few clinical studies on the effect of low level laser therapy on tooth movement. In a recent clinical trial, Sousa et al. [22] tested the influence of low-level laser irradiation to speed up the canine retraction in 13 patients. The irradiation protocol included an irradiation with a diode laser (780 nm/20 mW/10 s, 5 J/cm^2) for 3 days and the patients were followed up for 4 months. A significant increase in movement speed was found on the irradiated side compared to the contralateral control side without irradiation. No significant negative effects in bone and root resorption could be found. The same protocol (780 nm/20 mW/10 s, 5 J/cm^2) was used in a previous study of Cruz et al. [23] and showed similar results of a significant higher acceleration of canine retraction due to low level laser therapy. The same results were observed by Youssef et al. [see 29], who found a significant greater velocity in canine retraction using a low-level laser therapy (809 nm/100 mW/10 or 20 s/8 J per application). These results are not in agreement with the results found by Limpanichkul et al. [24, 25] who tested the effect of low level laser on orthodontic tooth movement in human patients and did not see any effect on the movement speed. In contrast to the first three studies, in this investigation a higher dose of laser (25 J/cm^2/2.3 J per point/18.4 J per tooth) was used. As described by Goulart et al. [25], higher doses of LLL could result in inhibitory effects on tooth movement and be the reason for these contrary results. Similar to human studies, diverse results are found in animal studies concerning the positive effect of laser therapy on the speed of tooth movement. Kawasaki and Shimizu [8] reported that low-energy laser therapy increased tooth movement. In accordance with these results, Fujita et al. [7] and Yamaguchi et al. [6] found an increase in tooth movement velocity. In contrast, Marquezan et al. [9] looked at the effect of two different laser protocols on the experimental tooth movement in rats and did not find an increase in tooth movement. After daily application, an increase in the number of osteoclasts could be found and the expression of immature collagen was inhibited. The same conclusion was drawn by Kim et al. [15] who saw a facilitation in reorganization of connective tissue in rats during tooth movement after low-level laser irradiation but no difference in the amount of tooth moment compared to the irradiated group. In accordance, Seifi et al. [26] did not find an effect on the speed of tooth movement in rabbits with pulsed or continuous laser application. The same results in a rat study were found by Gama et al. [27] who could not register an increased amount of tooth movement in rats after laser application. One of the reasons for these diverse results may be the amount of energy used in the different experiments. Goulart et al. [25] evaluated the effect of laser irradiation on the speed of orthodontic moment of canines in dogs. They found a positive effect with an acceleration of orthodontic tooth movement with a 5.25 J/cm^2 dosage, whereas the 35.0 J/cm^2 dosage resulted in a retarded movement.

Abi-Ramia et al. [28] investigated another effect of low-level laser therapy recently. The authors looked at the microscopic pulpal reactions resulting from orthodontic tooth movement in combination with a low-level laser therapy in a rat study. In literature there are controversial results of pulpal alterations described due to orthodontic tooth movement depending on the study design. Regarding the effect of low-level laser therapy on the pulp this study showed an increase in vascularization and the pulpal responses were restricted to the area underneath the region of orthodontic force and laser application. These results offer the conclusion that the laser therapy leads to an accelerated tissue repair during orthodontically induced tooth movement.

Conclusion and Future Perspectives

The literature review of the effects of low-level laser therapy in orthodontic therapy showed beneficial results concerning the reduction of the postadjustment pain as well as the influence on acceleration of tooth movement.

Clinical studies investigating the influence of low-level laser therapy on the pain due to the applied orthodontic force showed concordant results concluding that the initial pain after initiation of the orthodontic appliance could be reduced due to the effect of low-level laser therapy [18–21].

Regarding the effect of laser therapy on the amount of tooth movement there are controversial results in the literature. On the one hand, most of the studies are experimental or animal studies and only four clinical trials [22–24, 29] report on the effect on orthodontic tooth movement in humans. On the other hand, the laser devices as well as the irradiation protocols are not comparable in all cases. Consequently, there are authors that conclude that there is no acceleration on tooth movement seen due to the laser therapy

[9, 15, 24, 26, 27]. Others report a significant increase in the amount of tooth movement due to laser therapy [6–8, 22, 23, 29]. The reason for these diverse results is assumed to be the dosage of the applied laser. While low doses are associated with speeding up tooth movement, higher doses seem to have an inhibiting effect [25].

In conclusion, low-level laser therapy seems to have a high potential in improving orthodontic therapy regarding the patients comfort as well as reducing treatment time. Nevertheless, further studies are necessary to show results and help to find the right energy level and applying protocol to offer the most efficient support in orthodontic therapy. Compared to surgical techniques to speed up orthodontic treatment time this method combines an easy, noninvasive technique with the advantage of additional pain relieve rather than accelerating patients' stress by an additional invasive surgical intervention.

References

1 Yamasaki K, Miura F, Suda T: Prostaglandin as a mediator of bone resorption induced by experimental tooth movement in rats. J Dent Res 1980;59:1635–1642.

2 Kale S, Kocadereli I, Atilla P, Asan E: Comparison of the effects of 1,25-dihydroxycholecalciferol and prostaglandin E$_2$ on orthodontic tooth movement. Am J Orthod Dentofacial Orthop 2004;125:607–614.

3 Takano-Yamamoto T, Kawakami M, Kobayashi Y, Yamashiro T, Sakuda M: The effect of local application of 1,25-dihydroxycholecalciferol on osteoclast numbers in orthodontically treated rats. J Dent Res 1992;71:53–59.

4 Collins MK, Sinclair PM: The local use of vitamin D to increase the rate of orthodontic tooth movement. Am J Orthod Dentofacial Orthop 1988;94:278–284.

5 Verna C, Dalstra M, Melsen B: The rate and the type of orthodontic tooth movement is influenced by bone turnover in a rat model. Eur J Orthod 2000;22:343–352.

6 Yamaguchi M, Hayashi M, Fujita S, Yoshida T, Utsunomiya T, Yamamoto H, et al: Low-energy laser irradiation facilitates the velocity of tooth movement and the expressions of matrix metalloproteinase-9, cathepsin K, and alpha(v) beta(3) integrin in rats. Eur J Orthod 2010;32:131–139.

7 Fujita S, Yamaguchi M, Utsunomiya T, Yamamoto H, Kasai K: Low-energy laser stimulates tooth movement velocity via expression of RANK and RANKL. Orthod Craniofac Res 2008;11:143–155.

8 Kawasaki K, Shimizu N: Effects of low-energy laser irradiation on bone remodeling during experimental tooth movement in rats. Lasers Surg Med 2000;26:282–291.

9 Marquezan M, Bolognese AM, Araujo MT: Effects of two low-intensity laser therapy protocols on experimental tooth movement. Photomed Laser Surg 2010;28:757–762.

10 Ozawa Y, Shimizu N, Kariya G, Abiko Y: Low-energy laser irradiation stimulates bone nodule formation at early stages of cell culture in rat calvarial cells. Bone 1998;22:347–354.

11 Saito S, Shimizu N: Stimulatory effects of low-power laser irradiation on bone regeneration in midpalatal suture during expansion in the rat. Am J Orthod Dentofacial Orthop 1997;111:525–532.

12 Ninomiya T, Hosoya A, Nakamura H, Sano K, Nishisaka T, Ozawa H: Increase of bone volume by a nanosecond pulsed laser irradiation is caused by a decreased osteoclast number and an activated osteoblasts. Bone 2007;40:140–148.

13 Ninomiya T, Miyamoto Y, Ito T, Yamashita A, Wakita M, Nishisaka T: High-intensity pulsed laser irradiation accelerates bone formation in metaphyseal trabecular bone in rat femur. J Bone Miner Metab 2003;21:67–73.

14 Habib FA, Gama SK, Ramalho LM, Cangussu MC, Santos Neto FP, Lacerda JA, et al: Laser-induced alveolar bone changes during orthodontic movement: a histological study on rodents. Photomed Laser Surg 2010;28:823–830.

15 Kim YD, Kim SS, Kim SJ, Kwon DW, Jeon ES, Son WS: Low-level laser irradiation facilitates fibronectin and collagen type I turnover during tooth movement in rats. Lasers Med Sci 2010;25:25–31.

16 Tayer BH, Burek MJ: A survey of adults' attitudes toward orthodontic therapy. Am J Orthod 1981;79:305–315.

17 Oliver RG, Knapman YM: Attitudes to orthodontic treatment. Br J Orthod 1985;12:179–188.

18 Lim HM, Lew KK, Tay DK: A clinical investigation of the efficacy of low level laser therapy in reducing orthodontic postadjustment pain. Am J Orthod Dentofacial Orthop 1995;108:614–622.

19 Turhani D, Scheriau M, Kapral D, Benesch T, Jonke E, Bantleon HP: Pain relief by single low-level laser irradiation in orthodontic patients undergoing fixed appliance therapy. Am J Orthod Dentofacial Orthop 2006;130:371–377.

20 Fujiyama K, Deguchi T, Murakami T, Fujii A, Kushima K, Takano-Yamamoto T: Clinical effect of CO(2) laser in reducing pain in orthodontics. Angle Orthod 2008;78:299–303.

21 Seiryu M, Deguchi T, Fujiyama K, Sakai Y, Daimaruya T, Takano-Yamamoto T: Effects of CO2 laser irradiation of the gingiva during tooth movement. J Dent Res 2010;89:537–542.

22 Sousa MV, Scanavini MA, Sannomiya EK, Velasco LG, Angelieri F: Influence of low-level laser on the speed of orthodontic movement. Photomed Laser Surg 2011;29:191–196.

23 Cruz DR, Kohara EK, Ribeiro MS, Wetter NU: Effects of low-intensity laser therapy on the orthodontic movement velocity of human teeth: a preliminary study. Lasers Surg Med 2004;35:117–120.

24 Limpanichkul W, Godfrey K, Srisuk N, Rattanayatikul C: Effects of low-level laser therapy on the rate of orthodontic tooth movement. Orthod Craniofac Res 2006;9:38–43.

25 Goulart CS, Nouer PR, Mouramartins L, Garbin IU, de Fatima Zanirato Lizarelli R: Photoradiation and orthodontic movement: experimental study with canines. Photomed Laser Surg 2006;24:192–196.

26 Seifi M, Shafeei HA, Daneshdoost S, Mir M: Effects of two types of low-level laser wave lengths (850 and 630 nm) on the orthodontic tooth movements in rabbits. Lasers Med Sci 2007;22:261–264.

27 Gama SK, Habib FA, Monteiro JS, Paraguassu GM, Araujo TM, Cangussu MC, et al: Tooth movement after infrared laser phototherapy: clinical study in rodents. Photomed Laser Surg 2010;28(suppl 2):S79–S83.

28 Abi-Ramia LB, Stuani AS, Stuani MB, Mendes Ade M: Effects of low-level laser therapy and orthodontic tooth movement on dental pulps in rats. Angle Orthod 2010;80:116–122.

29 Youssef M, Ashkar S, Hamade E, Gutknecht N, Lampert F, Mir M: The effect of low-level laser therapy during orthodontic movement: a preliminary study. Lasers Med Sci 2008;23:27–33.

Susanne Chiari, MD, DMD
Department of Orthodontics, Bernhard Gottlieb University Clinic of Dentistry
Medical University of Vienna
Sensengasse 2a
AT–1190 Vienna (Austria)
E-Mail susanne.chiari@meduniwien.ac.at

Kantarci A, Will L, Yen S (eds): Tooth Movement. Front Oral Biol. Basel, Karger, 2016, vol 18, pp 124–129
DOI: 10.1159/000351907

A Comparison between Osteotomy and Corticotomy-Assisted Tooth Movement

Stephen L-K Yen

Center for Craniofacial Molecular Biology, Ostrow School of Dentistry of the University of Southern California and Childrens Hospital Los Angeles, Los Angeles, Calif., USA

Abstract

Osteotomies and corticotomies used in combination with orthodontic tooth movement can activate different bone responses that may be exploited to accelerate tooth movement. Segmental osteotomies around dental roots can create a tooth-bearing transport disk that may be distracted and positioned with orthodontic appliances and archwires. In difficult craniofacial repairs, alveolar segments can be guided into position with archwires and orthodontic mechanics. The corticotomy extending into the marrow space can activate bone injury repair mechanisms that accelerate bone turnover as the alveolar bone surrounding the dental roots transitions from a demineralization phase to a fibrous replacement phase and, finally, a mineralization phase. The controlled demineralization and replacement of alveolar bone provides a window of opportunity for roots to move though less dense bone prior to remineralization. Although the corticotomies and osteotomies are minor surgeries compared to orthognathic surgery, the goal of future research is to produce similar bone responses by using smaller surgeries or by eliminating the surgeries altogether.

Dentoalveolar surgery used in combination with orthodontic tooth movement has the potential of changing the biology of tooth movement and has been exploited to accelerate tooth movement, to perform difficult tooth movements and to alter the dental archform. Although the additional morbidity of surgery is an important consideration, these strategies can be very useful in patients who are already undergoing periodic surgeries such as patients with craniofacial anomalies. The following examples are presented as illustrations of these strategies which will be followed by a discussion on the differences between an osteomy vs. corticotomy approaches for altering tooth movement [1, 2]. The patient depicted in figure 1 had a horizontally impacted incisor facing the cleft site that could not be uprighted using routine orthodontic mechanics. Part of the problem is the uneven distribution of bone around the incisor following an alveolar bone graft. In order to simultaneously reposition the tooth and create bone in the wake of the tooth movement, a box osteotomy was performed in order to create a distraction site. After the distraction callus formed, the osteotomized segment was rapidly repositioned in two weeks. The vertical and

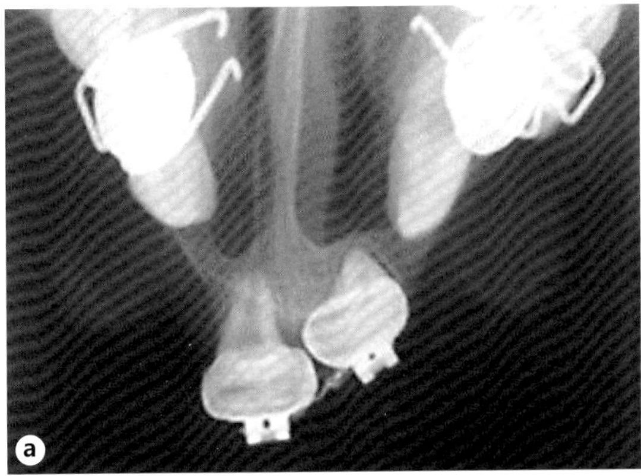

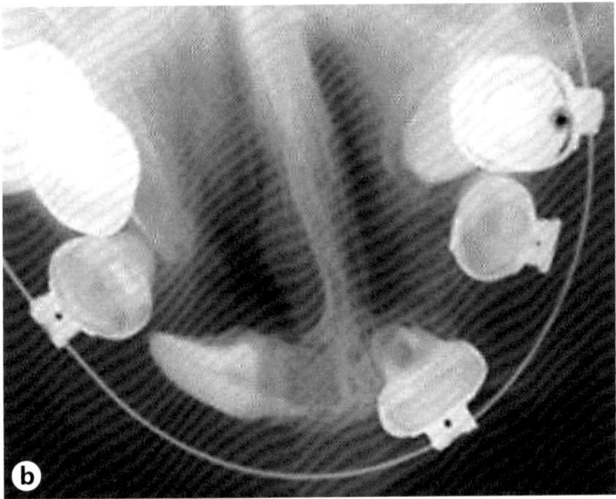

Fig. 1. Uprighting of a horizontally impacted incisor in a cleft site using osteotomy-assisted tooth movement. **a** Horizontal impaction in alveolar cleft site. **b** Tooth position 4 weeks after osteotomy and orthodontic correction of the bony segment.

horizontal cuts outlined but did not touch the dental root. At the interdental papilla regions, the vertical cut was incomplete leaving 5 mm of bone between the cut and the papilla. A modified osteotome made from a sharpened cement spatula was inserted into the cut sites to complete the segmental osteotomies [1]. The patient shown in figure 2 had a 21-mm anterior palatal fistula that was unsuccessfully treated with tongue flaps. In this case, osteotomies were placed around the roots of an ectopically erupted and palatally positioned tooth [2]. These cuts were used to create a transport disk that could be distracted along a track made from stainless steel wires spanning a lingual arch appliance. Using springs and wires to activate the distraction force, the transport disk was moved across the defect to close the anterior palatal fistula. After docking the transport disk, corticotomies were placed to expand the Y-shaped palatal arch into a U-shaped arch to allow the buccal plates to expand with the dental roots when elastic archwires were placed. This patient had a thick buccal cortical plate; a buccal onlay graft could have been used in combination with the corticotomy and arch expansion. Figure 3 shows an unrepaired facial cleft with vertically and laterally collapsed maxillary segments that had to be repositioned downward and outward like the lowering of a drawbridge that had halves positioned too closely and would hit unless the bases and hinges were also moving apart. In this case, LeFort I maxillary osteotomy segments were created that were moved into position with rectangular nickel-titanium archwires and springs that continuously prevented the segments from hitting and binding while the segments were lowered into position. After 3 weeks, the segments could be realigned into an arch form for an alveolar bone graft and orthodontic tooth alignment.

These cases illustrate how dentoalveolar surgery can be used to reshape the dental archform and solve difficult clinical problems in orthodontics and oral surgery. When Ilizarov [3, 4] described his animal and clinical research, one important tenet was the preservation of the bone marrow. His best outcomes in orthopedic lengthening of the long bones used corticotomies, not osteotomies. However, the alveolar bone at the level of the alveolar roots is different from long bones. Cortical bone can vary in bone thickness and density; the medullary space is not always clearly defined around the dental roots. Corticotomy-assisted tooth has been associated with regional accelerated phenomenon, a term coined by Frost [5, 6], for a process of accelerated bone remodeling during fracture repair. It is called 'regional' because the changes in bone turnover

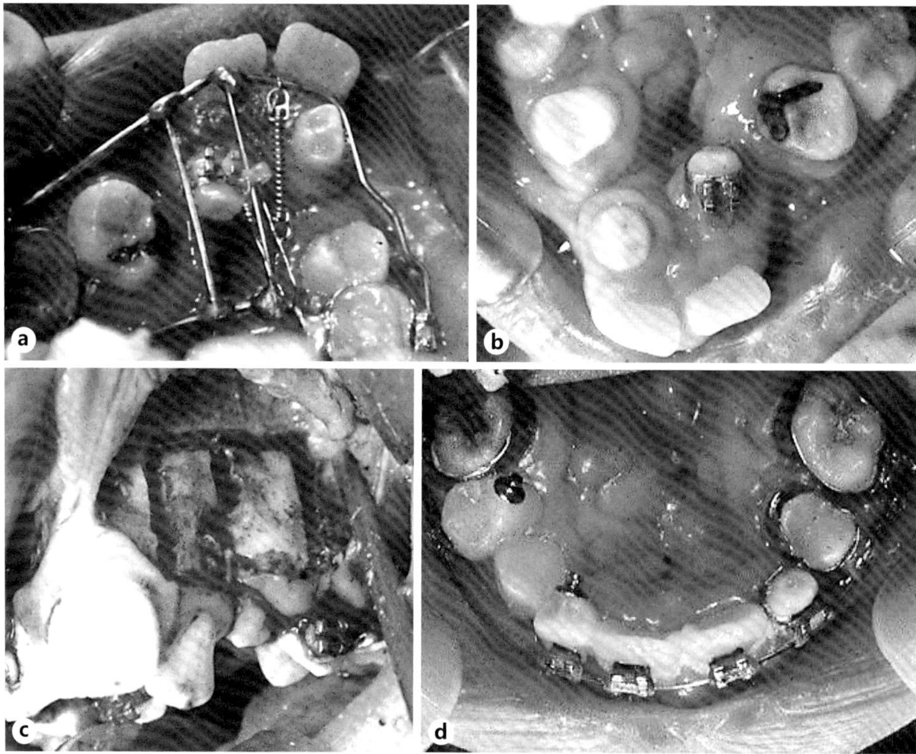

Fig. 2. Correction of an unusually large palatal fistula. Transport disk using alveolar segment containing palatal tooth. **a** Postdistraction correction of fistula. **b** Collapsed archform. **c** Corticotomies. **d** Widening of archform with corticotomies.

can also occur at sites distant from the fracture or corticotomy site. It is called 'acceleratory' because both bone resorption and bone formation processes are accelerated as part of the fracture and injury repair process [7].

The question of how alveolar bone responds to corticotomies and osteotomies is interesting because Ilizarov favored the use of corticotomies in the long bone yet the clinical evidence suggested a regional accelerated phenomenon (RAP) with corticotomy-assisted tooth movement. In orthodontics, RAP is thought to produce a temporary demineralization of bone around the dental roots that can be exploited for rapid tooth movement [8]. Once the alveolar bone is demineralized, the teeth can be rapidly moved through the demineralized matrix so that bone will remineralize around

the roots in their new positions. Some proponents use a bone graft to cover the buccal root, to ensure that there is bone around the roots after treatment and to maintain the width of the alveolar ridge. The corticotomy that extends into the marrow space is thought to be the mechanism for inducing the initial RAP response. The demineralization and remineralization steps of corticotomy-assisted tooth movement are rapid so there is a narrow window of time of about two to three months, that can allow for rapid tooth movement. The speed of tooth movement slows down to a routine treatment timetable after this window of opportunity closes. In practice, the number of appointments for orthodontic adjustments is the same only squeezed into a weekly rather than a monthly schedule during the postcorticotomy treatment period.

Yen

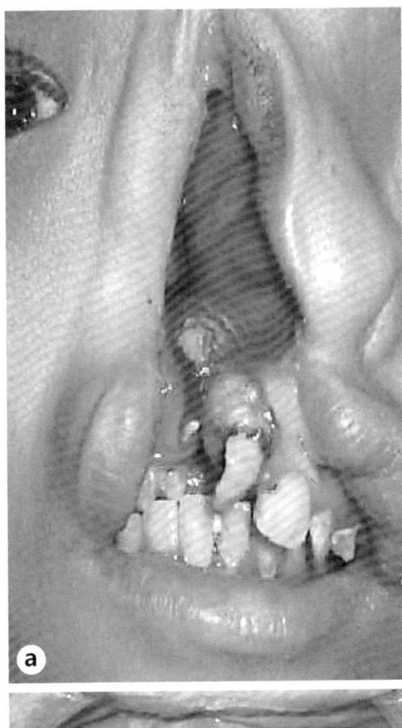

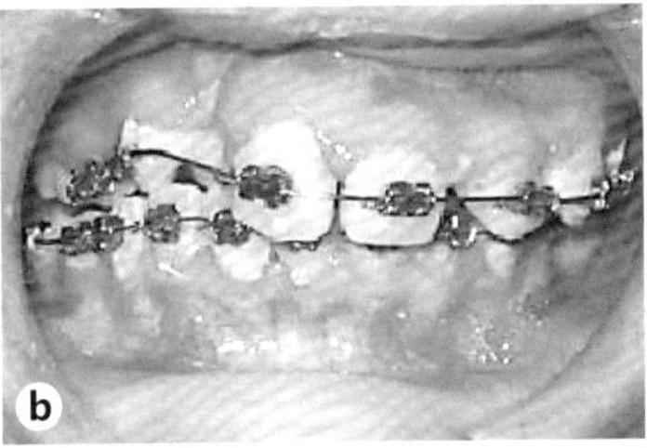

Fig. 3. a, b Use of LeFort 1 segmental osteotomy with orthodontic archwires to distract the cleft segments into an arch form and reposition the segment vertically.

Given the history and theories of corticotomy-assisted tooth movement, our laboratory studied whether alveolar bone would respond like the long bones in creating a distraction site or whether it would develop a RAP response that would demineralize bone around the dental roots. Using a rat model for tooth movement, corticotomy with and without tooth movement was compared to osteotomy with and without tooth movement as well as against tooth movement control animals [1]. This study was a prospective microCT investigation that collected that took initial, day 21 and 2 months' posttreatment microCTs on sedated animals. The corticotomy design was the same as the osteotomy; in the case of the osteotomy group the segment was freed with a micro-osteotome and then ligated to the host bone with wires. The continuous bony contact during the latency phase of treatment promoted the formation of a fracture callus. Tooth movement was initiated 3 days after surgery. The bone density of the experimental sites were compared to the uncut contra-lateral side. Each treatment group was measured for luminosity pixel count at three levels and five positions surrounding the dental root in the segment. The corticotomy groups showed loss of bone around the dental roots at day 21. The osteotomy groups showed a cut site and the creation of a distal distraction site when tooth movement forces were applied. The normal tooth movement control showed a slight but noticeable amount of demineralization around the dental roots, a milder form of RAP that is consistent with other reports on tooth movement and RAP. The overall change seen in these studies (fig. 4) was the creation of a distraction site with osteotomy-assisted tooth movement; RAP occurred with corticotomy-assisted tooth movement. It would appear that distraction osteogenesis at the dentoalveolar level should be performed with an osteotomy rather than a corticotomy to avoid concomitant loss of bone during the initial phase of RAP.

In corticotomy-assisted tooth movement, the tissue histology shows loss of bone and replacement with fibrous tissue at day 21 (fig. 5). The osteoclast count was the highest at day 3 then fell off by day 21. TGFβ_1, a marker for osteoblast differentiation, and VEGF, a marker for neovascularization, peaked at day 21 and leveled off during the consolidation stage [9]. The bone density measurements using SCANCO software showed that corticotomy treated groups showed continuous demineralization until day 21 and then complete remineralization after 2 months (fig. 6). This data led us to describe the corticotomy-assisted tooth movement in terms of three phases: an initial demineralization phase (day 3), followed by a fibrous replacement phase (day 21) and remineralization (3 months).

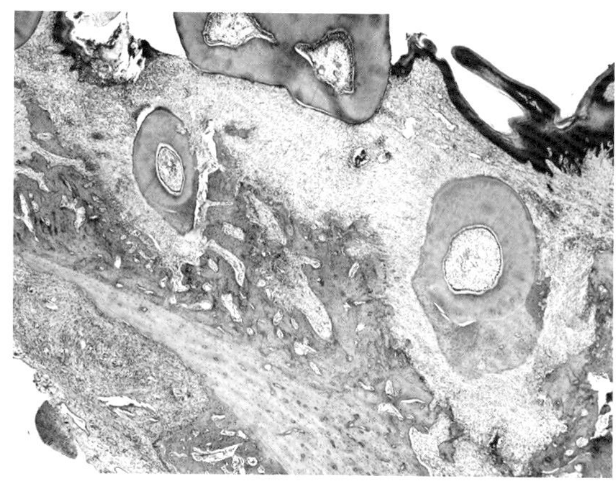

Fig. 4. MicroCT differences between osteotomy and corticotomy in rat tooth movement model. **a** Corticotomy-assisted tooth movement. **b** Osteotomy-assisted tooth movement

Fig. 5. Fibrous tissue replacement of bone around the dental roots as a mid-phase response in corticotomy-assisted tooth movement.

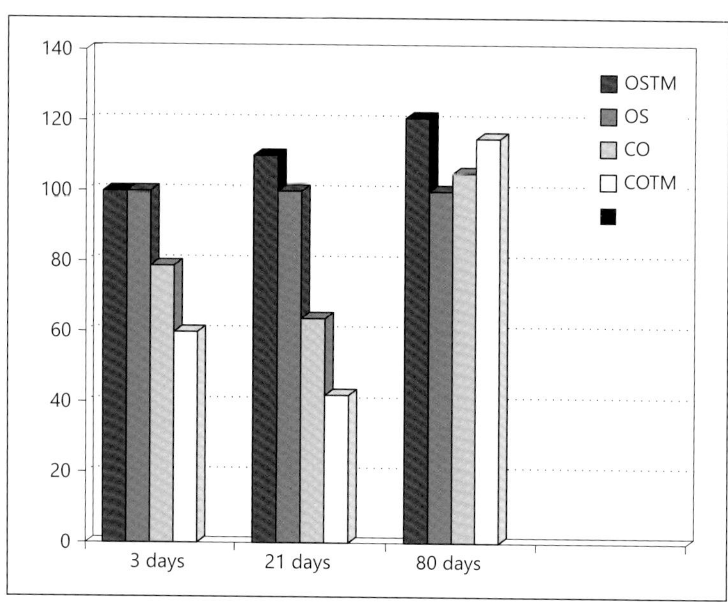

Fig. 6. Changes in bone volume compared to the uncut contralateral side (100%) using SCANCO bone histomorphometric software with microCT images of rat tooth movement with osteotomies alone (OS), osteotomies with tooth movement (OSTM), corticotomies alone (CO) and corticotomy-assisted tooth movement (COTM).

Yen

Both osteotomy and corticotomy can help accelerate tooth movement but the mechanisms may be different. With osteotomy-assisted tooth movement, there can be rapid repositioning of an osteotomized alveolar segment with archwires. With corticotomy-assisted tooth movement, the bone around the dental root demineralizes allowing for movement through the demineralized bone prior to remineralization. Both processes are part of bone repair and may overlap in response properties. For example, distraction osteogenesis could involve a RAP response under certain conditions.

During distraction osteogenesis, the center of the distraction site is fibrous with bone forming from the bony ends toward the fibrous center after the segments are stabilized during the consolidation phase. The actual distraction site may also show signs of both intramembranous bone formation with formation of primary bone and endochondral bone formation with islands of cartilage in the distraction site. Our laboratory performed studies that suggest that the stability of the distrac-

tion segments could be important in determining whether intramembranous or endochondral bone formation occurs. With less stable fixation, these conditions favor endochondral bone formation and the expression of sox 9, a marker for chondrogenesis in the distraction site. Instability in fracture repair shows similar changes in bone formation. Less stable fixation could result from loosened bone screws or too few screws for segment stability during the distraction procedure.

The current direction of research in corticotomy-assisted tooth movement is to produce the RAP response without the surgical intervention and eliminate the surgical morbidity. There are several promising approaches for recapitulating the RAP response by activating the cells involved in bone turnover by using lasers and LED lights. Further research is needed to confirm whether these approaches can produce the biological changes needed for clinical applications such as faster tooth movement, bone formation and changes in arch form.

References

1 Lee W, Karapetyan G, Moats R, Yamashita DD, Moon HB, Ferguson DJ, Yen S: Corticotomy-/osteotomy-assisted tooth movement microCTs differ. J Dent Res 2008;87:861–865.
2 Yen SL, Yamashita DD, Gross J, Meara JG, Yamazaki K, Kim TH, et al: Combining orthodontic tooth movement with distraction osteogenesis to close cleft spaces and improve maxillary arch form in cleft lip and palate patients. Am J Orthod Dentofacial Orthop 2005;127:224–232.
3 Ilizarov GA: The principles of the Ilizarov method. Bull Hosp Jt Dis 1988;56: 49–53.
4 Ilizarov GA: The tension-stress effect on the genesis and growth of tissues. Part I. The influence of stability of fixation. Clin Orthop Relat Res 1989;238:249–281.
5 Frost HM: The biology of fracture healing. An overview for clinicians. Part I. Clin Orthop Rel Res 1989;248:283–293.
6 Frost HM: The biology of fracture healing. An overview for clinicians. Part II. Clin Orthop Rel Res 1989;248:294–309.
7 Bogoch E, Gschwend N, Rahn B, Moran E, Perren S: Healing of cancellous bone osteotomy in rabbits. Part I. Regulation of bone volume and the regional acceleratory phenomenon in normal bone. J Orthop Res 1993;11:285–291.
8 Iino S, Sakoda S, Ito G, Nishimori T, Ikeda T, Miyawaki S: Acceleration of orthodontic tooth movement by alveolar corticotomy in the dog. Am J Orthod Dentofacial Orthop 2007;131:448.e1–e8.
9 Wang L, Lee W, Lei DL, Liu YP, Yamashita DD, Yen SL: Tissue responses in corticotomy- and osteotomy-assisted tooth movements in rats: histology and immunostaining. Am J Orthod Dentofacial Orthop 2009;136:770e1–770e11.

Stephen L-K Yen, DMD, PhD
Center for Craniofacial Molecular Biology
Ostrow School of Dentistry of the University of Southern California
2250 Alcazar Street, CSA 103
Los Angeles, CA 90033-9062 (USA)
E-Mail syen@usc.edu

Kantarci A, Will L, Yen S (eds): Tooth Movement. Front Oral Biol. Basel, Karger, 2016, vol 18, pp 130
DOI: 10.1159/000351910

Conclusion and Future Directions

Accelerated orthodontic tooth movement is not simply the outcome of an increased application of forces. Such an approach will only result in ankylosis and root resorption, arresting the migration of the teeth in the alveolar bone. Recognition of this critical notion has led researchers to investigate the biological basis of orthodontic treatment. A thorough understanding requires a holistic approach to the entire tissue architecture, its vascularization and neuronal regulation, the impact of hormones and age, and how biomechanics affect these processes. All these events happen in the most sophisticated organ system in mammalians where hard and soft tissues meet in an environment exposed to the largest number of species in a biofilm known to exist in humans. Needless to add, we are just scratching the surface of understanding this complex biology. Our goal in this volume was to present and discuss the recent advances in this field. This required an outstanding team of experts, who presented both the basic science concepts and their relationship with the clinical practice. It is our hope that our contribution will set the stage for future research and researchers, who would take the full advantage of this exciting era where high-throughput methods of assessment of biological processes will be incorporated into the clinical practice of accelerated orthodontics.

Alpdogan Kantarci, Cambridge, Mass.
Stephen Yen, Los Angeles, Calif.
Leslie A. Will, Boston, Mass.

Author Index

Subject Index